Essential Practices in Hospice and Palliative Medicine

Fifth Edition

Essential Practices in Hospice and Palliative Medicine
Fifth Edition

UNIPAC 5
COMMUNICATION AND TEAMWORK

Lara Michal Skarf, MD
Harvard Medical School
VA Boston Healthcare System
Boston, MA

Katie H. Stowers, DO
University of Texas Health Science Center San Antonio
San Antonio, TX

Andrew Thurston, MD
University of Pittsburgh
Pittsburgh, PA

Reviewed by
Katie Neuendorf, MD
Cleveland Clinic
Cleveland, OH

Edited by
Joseph W. Shega, MD
Vitas Healthcare
Miami, FL

Miguel A. Paniagua, MD FACP
University of Pennsylvania
Philadelphia, PA

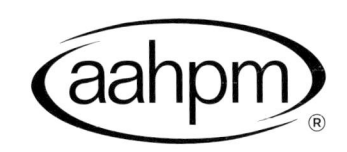

aahpm®

AMERICAN ACADEMY OF
HOSPICE AND PALLIATIVE MEDICINE

8735 W. Higgins Rd., Ste. 300
Chicago, IL 60631
aahpm.org | PalliativeDoctors.org

The information presented and opinions expressed herein are those of the editors and authors and do not necessarily represent the views of the American Academy of Hospice and Palliative Medicine. Any recommendations made by the editors and authors must be weighed against the healthcare provider's own clinical judgment, based on but not limited to such factors as the patient's condition, benefits versus risks of suggested treatment, and comparison with recommendations of pharmaceutical compendia and other medical and palliative care authorities.

Some discussions of pharmacological treatments in *Essential Practices in Hospice and Palliative Medicine* may describe off-label uses of drugs commonly used by hospice and palliative medicine providers. "Good medical practice and the best interests of the patient require that physicians use legally available drugs, biologics, and devices according to their best knowledge and judgment. If physicians use a product for an indication not in the approved labeling, they have the responsibility to be well informed about the product, to base its use on firm scientific rationale and on sound medical evidence, and to maintain records of the product's use and effects. Use of a marketed product in this manner *when the intent is the 'practice of medicine'* does not require the submission of an Investigational New Drug Application (IND), Investigational Device Exemption (IDE), or review by an Institutional Review Board (IRB). However, the institution at which the product will be used may, under its own authority, require IRB review or other institutional oversight" (US Food and Drug Administration, https://www.fda.gov/RegulatoryInformation/Guidances/ucm126486.htm, Updated January 25, 2016, Accessed May 17, 2017).

Published in the United States by the American Academy of Hospice and Palliative Medicine, 8735 W. Higgins Rd., Ste. 300, Chicago, IL 60631.

© 2017 American Academy of Hospice and Palliative Medicine
First edition published 1997
Second edition published 2003
Third edition published 2008
Fourth edition published 2012

All rights reserved, including that of translation into other languages. No part of this publication may be reproduced or transmitted in any form or by any means, electronic or mechanical, including photocopying, recording, or any information storage and retrieval system, without permission in writing from the copyright holder.

AAHPM Education Staff
Julie Bruno, Director, Education and Learning
Angie Forbes, Manager, Education and Learning
Kemi Ani, Manager, Education and Learning
Angie Tryfonopoulos, Coordinator, Education and Learning

AAHPM Editorial Staff
Jerrod Liveoak, Senior Editorial Manager
Bryan O'Donnell, Managing Editor
Andie Bernard, Assistant Editor
Tim Utesch, Graphic Designer
Jean Iversen, Copyeditor

ISBN 978-1-889296-25-8

Contents

Tables vii
Figures ix
Acknowledgments xi
Communication 1
    Effective Communication 1
    Impacts of Clinician Communication 3
    Communication and Hospice and Palliative Medicine 5
Barriers to Effective Communication 9
    Cultural Barriers 9
    Addressing Cultural Barriers 11
    Psychological Barriers 12
    Listening Barriers 14
    Organizational/System Barriers 16
    Language Barriers 16
    Other Barriers 18
Strategies for Effective Communication 19
    Understand Nonverbal Communication 19
    Encourage Patients to Talk and Listen to What They Say 20
    Ask Before Telling 21
    Respond with Empathy 21
    Manage Uncertainty 24
    Use Appropriate Humor 26
Communicating Serious News 29
    General Guidelines for Communicating Serious News 30
    A Six-Step Protocol for Communicating Serious News 32
    Special Considerations 45
Communicating to Achieve a Shared Decision 49
    Clinical Decisions 49
Communicating Prognosis 57
    Gauging Prognostic Awareness 57
    Discussing Prognosis 58
    Denial and the Patient 60
    Denial and the Family 61
    Troubleshooting Prognosis 62
    Communicating with Loved Ones 65

    Family Systems Theory 66
    The Family Life Cycle. 67
    Family Interaction Models 67
    Family Subsystems 68
    Family Responses to Terminal Illness and Death 70
    Facilitating Family Conferences 71
    Roadmaps for Family Conferences 73

Selected Communication Issues. 81
    Confidentiality. 81
    Communication with Colleagues and Referring Providers 82
    Communication with Patients with Dementia and Their Caregivers. 84
    Communicating with Young Children of Dying Patients. 87
    Communication with the Dying Patient 87
    Communication Strategies During Telehealth Encounters 88
    Limited English Proficiency. 90
    Communication with Patients Who Are Lesbian, Gay, Bisexual, and Transgender 90
    Communication Surrounding Organ Donation 93

The Interdisciplinary Team 95
    Suffering and the Interdisciplinary Team Approach to Care 95
    The Function of the Team 96
    Requirements for a Hospice IDT. 97
    General Characteristics of the IDT 97
    Building the Team. 99
    Threats to Team Performance 111

Coping with Stress 117
    Difficult Encounters 117
    Burnout 117
    Stress-Management Strategies 118

Summary. 125
References 127
Index 145

Tables

Table 1.	Six Core Components of Patient-Centered Communication	3
Table 2.	General Communication Guidelines	7
Table 3.	Common Barriers to Effective Communication	10
Table 4.	Effective Communication Strategies	22
Table 5.	Ask-Tell-Ask	24
Table 6.	Strategies to Manage Uncertainty	25
Table 7.	Patients' Preferences When Physicians Communicate Serious News	30
Table 8.	SPIKES Protocol for Communicating Serious News	33
Table 9.	Statements for Eliciting Patient Perspective	35
Table 10.	NURSE Mnemonic: Ways to Verbally Address Emotions	39
Table 11.	SAVE	39
Table 12.	Strategies to Display Empathy	41
Table 13.	Identifying Goals, Values, and Preferences	51
Table 14.	REMAP	52
Table 15.	Sample Statements for Shared Decision Making	53
Table 16.	Strategies for Responding to Requests for Nondisclosure of Information	63
Table 17.	"Hope and Worry" and "I Wish" Statements	64
Table 18.	Characteristics of Open and Closed Family Systems	69
Table 19.	Communication and Counseling Techniques for Physicians During Family Conferences	74
Table 20.	Exploring Faith in a Family Conference	76
Table 21.	A Method for Optimizing Communication Between the Hospice and Palliative Medicine Consultant and a Consulting Physician	85
Table 22.	Tips for Effective Telemedicine Communication	89
Table 23.	Tips for Using an Interpreter	91
Table 24.	Communication with Nonheterosexual Individuals	92
Table 25.	Palliative Care Needs of Nonheterosexual Individuals	93
Table 26.	The Interdisciplinary Team: Description, Advantages, and Disadvantages	98
Table 27.	Developmental Phases of Interdisciplinary Healthcare Teams	99
Table 28.	Characteristics of Effective Interdisciplinary Teams	101
Table 29.	Skills of Effective Leaders	103
Table 30.	Decision-Making Methods	109
Table 31.	Common Problems and Barriers to Effective Teamwork	111
Table 32.	Symptoms of Dysfunctional Teams	113
Table 33.	Qualities of Effective Feedback	116

Table 34.	Factors Associated with Stress Overload Among Physicians	119
Table 35.	Signs and Symptoms of Stress Overload Among Physicians	120
Table 36.	Strategies to Manage Stress	121
Table 37.	Suggested Self-Care and Self-Awareness Workplace Practices	122
Table 38.	Training for Effective Communication	125
Table 39.	Curricular Resources for Teaching Communication Skills	126

Figures

Figure 1. Six Core Components of Patient-Centered Communication .4
Figure 2. Shared Decision-Making Continuum 54
Figure 3. A Model for the Team Decision-Making Process 108

Acknowledgments

AAHPM is deeply grateful to all who have participated in the development of this component of the *Essential Practices in Hospice and Palliative Medicine* self-study program. The expertise of the editors, contributors, and reviewers involved in the current and previous editions of the Essentials series has ensured the value of its content to our field.

AAHPM extends special thanks to the authors of previous editions of this volume: Toby C. Campbell, MD, Gordon J. Wood, MD, C. Porter Storey, Jr., MD FACP FAAHPM, and Carol F. Knight, EdM; the authors of the *UNIPAC 5 amplifire* online learning module, Yuya Hagiwara, MD, Susan Nathan, MD, and Katie H. Stowers, DO; the pharmacist reviewer for this edition of the *Essentials* series, Jennifer Pruskowski, PharmD; and the many professionals who volunteered their time and expertise to review the content and test this program in the field—Joe Rotella, MD MBA HMDC FAAHPM, Stuart J. Farber, MD, Joseph W. Shega, MD, Stacie K. Levine, MD, Joshua Hauser, MD, John W. Finn, MD FAAHPM, Walter B. Forman, MD, Rev. Milton W. Hay, DMin, Michael E. Frederich, MD FAAHPM, Barbara M. Henley, LMSW ACP, Gerald H. Holman, MD FAAFP, Rev. Charles Meyer, MDiv MS, Terry C. Muck, PhD, Eli N. Perencevich, DO, Charles G. Sasser, MD, Julia L. Smith, MD, and Bradley Stuart, MD.

Essential Practices in Hospice and Palliative Medicine was originally published in 1998 in six volumes as the *UNIPAC* self-study program. The first four editions of this series, which saw the addition of three new volumes, were created under the leadership of C. Porter Storey, Jr., MD FACP FAAHPM, who served as author and editor. AAHPM is proud to acknowledge Dr. Storey's commitment to and leadership of this expansive and critical resource, and the Academy's gratitude for his innumerable contributions cannot be overstated.

Continuing Medical Education

Continuing medical education credits are available, and Maintenance of Certification credits may be available, to users who complete the amplifire online learning module that has been created for each volume of *Essential Practices in Hospice and Palliative Medicine,* available for purchase from aahpm.org.

Communication

To ask physicians and patients to get to know themselves and each other better through conversation will encounter resistance. What has been true for the evolution of mankind has been equally true for the progress of medicine: We have spared no effort to make better tools but we have paid little attention to learning how to communicate better with one another.[1]

—Jay Katz

Almost invariably, the act of communication is an important part of therapy; occasionally it is the only constituent. It usually requires greater thought and planning than a drug prescription, and unfortunately it is commonly administered in sub-therapeutic doses.[2]

—Robert Buckman

In general, the most common problems are caused by relatively simple errors—faults in common courtesy, failures in listening or in acknowledging the patient's needs.[3]

—Robert Buckman

Studies have repeatedly shown that thorough histories provide 70% to 80% of the information needed to make most diagnoses, with physical examination, laboratory, and radiographic findings contributing the rest.[2,3] Effective communication is essential to elicit adequate information about the patient's physical, emotional, social, and spiritual concerns.

The goal of any physician-patient interaction is to establish and maintain an effective working relationship that promotes healing and mutual trust.[4] Effective communication is critical to promote this physician-patient relationship and is itself a therapeutic tool[5] and is considered the foundation of excellent patient care.[6] As a result, communication is now recognized as an important physician skill.[5,7,8]

Effective Communication

A growing body of medical literature provides guidance and best practices for effective communication during medical encounters.[7] Multiple organizations advocate the importance of communication that seeks to understand and incorporate an individual patient's unique values and perspectives into medical decision making. This type of communication is referred to as patient-centered[5,7] or relationship-centered communication.[9]

Patient-Centered Communication

The term patient-centered communication in relation to medical encounters emerged following the Institute of Medicine's 2001 pronouncement that medical care should become more patient centered. In this context, *patient-centered care* was defined as care that is more responsive to patient needs and perspectives, with patient values guiding decision making.[10] Precise definitions of patient-centered communication have varied over the years, but the common core components have remained the same. Patient-centered communication should

- elicit and understand patient perspectives (concerns, ideas, expectations, needs, feelings, and functioning)
- understand the patient within his or her unique psychosocial and cultural contexts
- reach a shared understanding of patient problems and the treatments that are concordant with patient values.[5]

Relationship-Centered Communication

Relationship-centered care is a framework that acknowledges that all illness and care occur in relationship to one's self and others. The Pew-Fetzer Task Force on Advancing Psychosocial Health Education, which convened in 1992 to bridge healthcare delivery systems and public health, described *relationship-centered care* as including relationships beyond the patient-physician relationship and defined it as care in which all participants appreciate the importance of their relationships with one another.[9]

Relationship-centered care is founded upon four principles:

1. Relationships in health care ought to include the personhood of the participants.
2. Affect and emotion are important components of these relationships.
3. All healthcare relationships occur in the context of reciprocal influence.
4. The formation and maintenance of genuine relationships in health care is morally valuable.

As a result, relationship-centered communication is a unique product of the participants and the context in which the conversation takes place. Quality relationship-centered communication is evaluated on how it further contributes to building the relationship between patient and provider.[9] While in many ways similar to patient-centered communication, relationship-centered communication emphasizes the importance of a strong and meaningful relationship between patient and provider in providing effective communication.

Patients today desire a care experience that is relationship centered and view communication between patient and physician as a two-way conversation. A recent study found that more than 80% of respondents expected their physician to listen to them, and more than half preferred that their physician elicit their goals and concerns.[11] This same study showed that patients prefer to be included in medical decisions, with a majority indicating a preference for physicians to share all treatment options, not just those recommended by the physician.[11]

Shared Decision Making

> *No single right decision exists for how the life of health and illness should be lived. . . . Physicians and patients [each] bring their own vulnerabilities to the decision-making process. Both are authors and victims of their own individual conflicting motivations, interests, and expectations. Identity of interests cannot be presumed. It can only be established through conversation.*[1]
>
> —Jay Katz

To achieve this patient-centered standard, physicians are faced with a dual agenda when making medical decisions in practice. Physicians must not only consider that which is medically appropriate but also that which is acceptable to the individual being treated. The physician must attend to both agendas, skillfully navigating and resolving discrepancies to achieve a mutually acceptable and medically appropriate care plan.[7] This is considered "shared decision making" and has become the "pinnacle" of patient-centered care in medical practice.[10]

General Components of Effective Communication

The National Cancer Institute identifies six core components of patient-centered communication that contribute to effective communication (**Table 1** and **Figure 1**).[5] These components are not intended to be hierarchical or independent. Instead, the components overlap and interact such that some components predominate depending on the context of the conversation. The Strategies for Effective Communication section (pages 19-27) provides practical tips and tools for applying these components of effective communication in practice.

Impacts of Clinician Communication

Benefits of Effective Communication

The increased emphasis on effective communication is grounded in a growing body of literature demonstrating beneficial clinical outcomes for patients and families as well as providers. Interventions that improve clinician communication have been linked to favorable patient outcomes such as improved quality of life, mood, and survival[12-14]; a preference for less aggressive care as death approaches[15,16]; and improved adherence to therapeutic regimens.[17]

Communication interventions also benefit families and surrogates. They have been shown to improve understanding of patient goals[15,16] and result in better caregiver psychological adjustment.[12,16] Effective communication also influences decision-making outcomes such as conflict[18] and error rates,[19] which, as a result, has been shown to decrease malpractice litigation.[20] Effective communication has been shown to favorably affect resource outcomes, including decreasing length of stay in the intensive care unit[15,18] and costs.[21] Interventions to improve clinician communication have also been shown to provide benefit to providers by increasing empathy and decreasing burnout. Specifically, communication training has been shown to decrease emotional exhaustion[22,23] and depersonalization[23,24] and increase a sense of personal achievement among clinicians.[23]

Table 1. Six Core Components of Patient-Centered Communication[5]

Fostering healing relationships
Exchanging information
Responding to emotions
Managing uncertainty
Making shared decisions
Enabling patient self-management

Figure 1. Six Core Components of Patient-Centered Communication

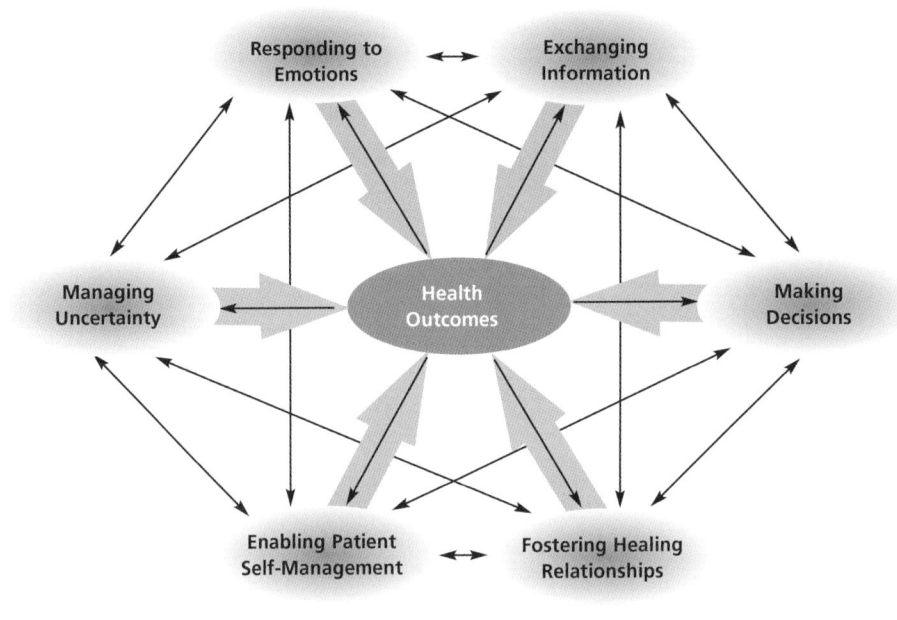

The six core functions of patient-clinician communication overlap and interact to produce communication that can affect important health outcomes.

From Patient-Centered Communication in Cancer Care: Promoting Health and Reducing Suffering *(Figure 2.1), by Epstein RM, Street RL, Jr., Bethesda, MD, National Cancer Institute, NIH Publication No. 07-6225, 2007.*[5]

Burdens of Ineffective Communication

Healthcare provider communication often fails to meet the needs of patients and families.[16] The potential impact of poor communication is dire. Communication breakdowns have been shown to result in the provision of poor medical care.[7] Unsatisfactory physician-patient communication has been linked to increases in malpractice claims.[20] At the end of life, adverse mental health sequelae; late hospice referrals; and more aggressive, unwanted, life-prolonging care are all potential consequences of ineffective communication.[16]

Patient and Family Satisfaction

Finding a correlation between communication and satisfaction has historically been problematic, with studies showing modest but inconsistent improvement in patient satisfaction with the implementation of communication skills training.[25] Many determinants of satisfaction are difficult to measure or are out of the medical community's control and often may reflect other experiences not impacted by communication.[15]

The Centers for Medicare and Medicaid Services (CMS) requirement to publicly report patient experience scores has led to the ability to measure patient satisfaction with communication. A 2016 study of 3,488 physicians showed that participation in a full-day training course in relationship-centered communication positively influenced patient satisfaction scores.[23] Patient satisfaction may depend more on the perception of adequate information sharing and emotional support than on the amount of time a physician spends with a patient. When a physician sits down, this simple act increases patient satisfaction.[26] Studies of patients with cancer indicate that patient satisfaction improves when physicians address their concerns and provide information with warmth, interest, and empathy.

Certain measures, such as discussing advance directives[27] and fostering trust, have been consistently linked to increased overall patient satisfaction with one's physicians. Patients report greater trust in their physician if they feel they have been listened to, receive as much information as they want, are told what to do if things change, are involved in decision making to the extent they desire, and spend as much time with their physician as they want.[28] Practical skills, such as using metaphors and analogies to help explain difficult topics, have been linked to improved patient ratings of communication.[29]

Family satisfaction with communication has also been examined, mostly in the intensive care unit setting. One potential technique to improve satisfaction is to allow a family more time to speak. One study found this technique leads to higher family satisfaction with physician communication.[30] Other factors that lead to higher satisfaction are assuring nonabandonment, providing comfort, supporting family decisions,[31] and giving complete information.[32]

Communication and Hospice and Palliative Medicine

Effective communication is recognized as one of the key skills of palliative care physicians and a primary task of hospice and palliative care organizations.[33-35] Communication and decision making have been found to be critical factors in achieving a "good death."[36] Effective communication is of such importance at the end of a patient's life that it should be considered a formal medical and psychosocial intervention that needs to be researched and employed like any other medical intervention.[37] Communication is often considered to be the hospice and palliative medicine physician's "core procedure." Several sets of quality indicators identify communication and decision making as primary quality indicators for end-of-life care.[38-42] Although the importance of effective communication skills is accepted in the field, validated communication assessment measures are challenging to develop and are thus lacking. Therefore, communication and decision-making indicators are not directly included in all quality measurement tools. "Measuring What Matters: Top 10 Quality Indicator Set" developed by AAHPM and the Hospice and Palliative Nurses Association includes several validated communication and decision-making indicators; however, the report notes the absence of any validated and universally accepted assessment tools in the areas of social and cultural aspects of care and does not include these indicators due to the lack of scientific evidence and insufficient documentation for feasible abstraction.[43]

Hospice and palliative medicine physicians must demonstrate competence in key communication tasks, such as listening to patients' life stories and understanding and honoring their meanings.[44] Without effective communication, physicians may inadvertently exacerbate a patient's suffering by focusing only on the disease and ignoring emotional, spiritual, and social concerns.

In hospice and palliative care settings, the three most common elements of communication are transmitting medical information, engaging in therapeutic dialogue, and sharing decision making with patients and their families.[45] Transmitting medical information often involves sharing bad news with patients and families,[46] while therapeutic dialogue involves exploring how the patient and family are coping with the illness and attempting to understand their deepest concerns. Communicating the goal of shared decision making allows the patient's values and preferences and the physician's clinical knowledge and expertise to lead the two parties to a joint decision for care.[47]

Physicians generally include both medical information and therapeutic dialogue in any patient interview; however, the mix often changes during the course of a terminal illness. Transmitting information initially may predominate, but therapeutic dialogue often becomes much more important as the patient's condition deteriorates and death approaches. Throughout the course of a terminal illness, patients and their family members look to physicians not only for knowledge and technical skill but also for guidance, reassurance, hope, meaning, and compassionate understanding. The ability to communicate effectively and compassionately is essential because it contributes to the creation and maintenance of therapeutic, interpersonal relationships and the exchange of information during assessments and decision making.[48]

For practitioners of hospice and palliative medicine, the ability to communicate compassionately is particularly important because the patient-physician relationship most often involves a person with serious illness who may be frail, frightened, and vulnerable and a physician who possesses specialized knowledge about the illness and its trajectory, along with its symptoms and effective palliative treatments. The patient's vulnerability, coupled with the intimacy of the physician-patient relationship, necessitates stringent ethical demands on both parties. Honest and compassionate communication is at the foundation of a trusting relationship.[49]

Several highly regarded sets of guidelines for effective communication have been published.[16,50-52] **Table 2** features general communication guidelines in hospice and palliative medicine.

Table 2. General Communication Guidelines

Effective palliative medicine depends on honest communication from patients about their symptoms, preferences, and concerns and honest communication from physicians about the patient's disease, prognosis, and likely benefits and burdens of treatments.[53]

Honest, compassionate, ongoing communication is a central component of hospice and palliative medicine. Communication increases the patient's and family's sense of control and self-worth, and it helps establish healing bonds among patients, families, physicians, and other healthcare professionals.

The sense of being heard is a crucial healing agent for dying patients and their family members.[54] Poor communication contributes to suffering because it can exacerbate the patient and family's sense of isolation, helplessness, and anxiety.

Although specific techniques can improve communication, the essence of true communication is the ability to enter into therapeutic relationships with mutual regard, respect, warmth, genuineness, and unconditional acceptance. Such relationships are characterized by empathic listening, attentiveness, presence, dialogue, and acknowledgment.[55]

Because stress, pain, and anxiety interfere with a patient's and family's ability to hear and retain information, it is important to alleviate distressing symptoms as soon as possible, establish therapeutic relationships, and repeat information as often as necessary.

Involving an interdisciplinary healthcare team helps patients and families voice their experiences through story, art, music, poetry, biography, and ritual.[56]

Barriers to Effective Communication

Among interpersonal relationships, the doctor-patient relation is one of the most complex ones. It involves interaction between individuals in non-equal positions, is often non-voluntary, concerns issues of vital importance, is therefore emotionally laden and requires close cooperation.[57]

—Samario Chaitchik, et al.

Communication barriers through the course of serious illness are widespread yet unique to each patient-physician relationship, making generalization difficult.[58] **Table 3** lists common barriers.

Cultural Barriers

Culture refers to the innate behaviors, beliefs, and values held important to a person; it is defined by more than ethnicity, race, or religion and is shaped by the vast experiences and societal influences in a person's life. Culture provides a framework for an individual to interpret the world, thus the same words spoken to two different people can be interpreted very differently. Cultural differences can impact communication; each culture has a unique set of norms that acts as the framework for integrating new data, rules about proper behavior that affect verbal and nonverbal communication, and expectations related to displays of emotion.[61] Because cultural beliefs, values, and expectations about health care affect communication among physicians, patients, and family members,[62,63] physicians must be sensitive to the cultural barriers discussed below.[46,59]

Unrealistic Expectations of the Healthcare System
In industrialized countries, highly publicized reports of alleged medical breakthroughs and miraculous cures contribute to the public's unrealistic expectations about health and illness. Despite receiving a diagnosis of a serious, debilitating, or incurable illness, patients may still expect to return to good health.[64]

Changes in Societal Values
Cultural values surrounding productivity, youth, physical attractiveness, and material wealth cannot help but affect a patient's sense of self-worth when diagnosed with a serious illness. Society's deepest values also inform public policy on the availability and quality of care for seriously or terminally ill patients.

Religion and Spirituality
In the United States increased secularization and religious pluralism contribute to uncertainty among physicians when discussing serious illness with patients. Religious and spiritual beliefs can greatly influence a patient's perspective and preferences for care. A patient may be unwilling to discuss prognosis or engage in end-of-life planning because of the belief that the nature and timing of death can only be determined by a "higher power." Some end-of-life practices

Table 3. Common Barriers to Effective Communication[46,59,60]

Cultural barriers	Unrealistic expectations of the healthcare system Changes in societal values Changing role of religion Lack of experience with death and dying Cultural beliefs regarding disclosure of information Trust Family involvement in decision making Filial responsibility
Psychological barriers	Patient's fears of • dying • physical symptoms • psychological effects • treatments • financial matters • changes in roles Family's fears of • physical care and emotional distress • financial repercussions • role changes Physician's fears of • sympathetic pain • expressing emotion • eliciting an emotional response • doing harm • illness or death • lack of knowledge • lack of communication skills training
Listening barriers	Judgment and evaluation Assumption and certainty Limited attention span
Organizational/system barriers	Healthcare environment and reimbursement issues Lack of motivation and standards of performance Lack of organizational support Disparities in access and information
Language barriers	Medical language Limited language skills Vocabulary

(eg, withholding and discontinuing life-sustaining therapies) may not be acceptable or may be considered to impact the patient's afterlife (see *UNIPAC 2*).[65]

Physicians can no longer assume that patients share similar beliefs about death and immortality, even when they belong to the same religious tradition. For this reason, it is important to elicit the beliefs and traditions important to each individual patient, avoiding assumptions and generalization.

Lack of Experience with Death and Dying
In the United States there is a general trend toward deaths occurring in institutions rather than in homes, which means fewer people have witnessed death. When distressing symptoms are adequately controlled, witnessing the death of another person may be reassuring rather than worrisome, as evidenced by decreased anxiety about dying among hospice patients who observed the peaceful death of another hospice patient.[66]

Cultural Beliefs About Disclosure of Information
Communication can be complicated by important cultural differences regarding disclosure of diagnosis and prognosis. Research indicates major regional differences in physicians' and patients' attitudes and beliefs about communication throughout the course of serious illness.[67-70] Although current trends in the United States favor more disclosure, the international norm is for less disclosure.[27] Cultural beliefs in the United States about disclosure vary widely. In a study of 800 senior citizens in the United States, 90% of those of European and African descent claimed they would want to know about a terminal diagnosis. In contrast, 65% of respondents of Mexican descent and fewer than 50% of respondents of Native American and Korean descent reported they would want to know about a terminal diagnosis.[71]

Trust
Many cultures in the United States have been subject to inequities in care. This can engender a lack of trust in the medical system and adversely affect physician-patient communication.

Family Involvement in Decision Making
In many cultures the family makes all decisions for the patient so that she or he is not burdened while ill. Cultures that have a significant predilection for family-centered decision making include but are not limited to Korean American, Hispanic, and African American.[72,73]

Filial Responsibility
Many cultures, especially those rooted in Asia, promote the expectation that children will care for their parents. Discussion about nursing home or hospice care can pose a threat to this cultural expectation, creating a barrier to effective communication.[74]

Addressing Cultural Barriers
Physicians should facilitate open inquiry about the barriers discussed above to effectively communicate in a multicultural environment. Using open-ended questions to discern individual

perceptions of illness, decision-making preferences, views on illness, and perspectives on death and dying is important to overcome these cultural barriers. Asking "What should I know about you (or your loved one) to help me provide you with the best care?" is an effective way to initiate discussion without assumptions that allows the patient to guide the subsequent conversation to what he or she feels is the most important. Asking "Are you at peace?" or "Are you (or is your loved one) a spiritual or religious person?" often can be an effective introduction to a discussion of spirituality.[75] Patients prefer a nonjudgmental, patient-centered approach to cultural issues that is integrated with the rest of their care.[76] An open dialogue and subsequent attempts to acknowledge and accommodate any differences can often circumvent major obstacles.[74] Partnering with chaplains and community spiritual leaders can help improve communication and care.

Psychological Barriers
Patient Fears
Patients with serious illness are likely to fear the effects of the illness and the process of dying more than death itself. Fears often focus on uncontrolled symptoms, increased dependency, the sense of becoming a burden to family members and friends, inability to cope, dementia, abandonment, side effects of treatments, existential concerns, and financial losses.[77,78] Effective symptom control, adequate information, and ongoing emotional support help restore dignity and alleviate anxiety, depression, and desire for hastened death. Specifically, a multidisciplinary team approach has been shown to improve chronic obstructive pulmonary disease patients' sense of dignity, as well as depression and anxiety.[79] Specific interventions such as the Managing Cancer and Living Meaningfully (CALM) protocol—a brief, manualized, individual psychotherapeutic intervention—have demonstrated decreased anxiety about death and improved spiritual and emotional well-being for patients with cancer.[80] Meaning-centered group psychotherapy improved spiritual well-being and quality of life and decreased depression, hopelessness, desire for hastened death, and physical symptom distress for cancer patients.[81] Finally, a patient's need to occasionally avoid active discussion of their fears of death and dying also should be honored.

Family Fears
Family members often fear that they will be unable to provide the necessary physical care for their loved one. They may also doubt their ability to tolerate the emotional distress that might accompany the many losses that accumulate during the course of a serious illness, especially at the end of life. Financial concerns also are common. Thirty-one percent of families in the United States lose all or most of their savings during the course of a patient's terminal illness.[82] In addition, when one family member becomes seriously ill, other family members must adapt to changing roles. Assuming new roles is challenging and frightening, particularly when the illness necessitates unwelcome changes.[83]

Physician Fears

Fear of Being Changed

When physicians develop therapeutic relationships with patients, they rarely emerge unchanged. Attempting to truly understand a patient's point of view without making judgments may challenge the physician's long-held beliefs, which can be frightening.[41] However, physicians with the courage to risk being influenced by a patient's insights are likely to experience personal and professional growth.[84]

Fear of Expressing Emotion

Physicians may underestimate the amount of emotional distress they are likely to experience in the presence of someone who is suffering. When faced with a patient's life-threatening diagnosis, physicians may feel helpless or out of control. Because they are trained to conceal their feelings of irritation, panic, sorrow, and uncertainty, they may believe that good physicians never experience or express any emotion other than calm certitude. This myth is particularly harmful to those physicians providing care to people who are seriously ill. Patients rarely criticize physicians whose eyes tear up with emotion when sharing serious news. Acknowledging sympathetic pain among colleagues helps physicians cope with feelings of personal inadequacy and guilt generated by the myth that competent physicians are immune to a patient's suffering. Unless acknowledged, cumulative grief from personal and professional losses may result in emotional distance from patients.[85]

Fear of Eliciting an Emotional Response

When hearing information about a serious or life-threatening condition, patients and family members may experience shock, anger, or disbelief. They are likely to cry. Physicians, especially those who lack training in hospice and palliative medicine, may fear these normal reactions.[86,87] Anticipating emotional reactions can help physicians guide patients and families through the process of dealing with difficult news.[88,89]

Fear of Doing Harm

Physicians may fear doing harm to patients by exploring distressing events. However, a growing body of literature suggests these concerns may be unfounded. More information does not tend to increase worry,[90] and end-of-life discussions have not been shown to increase patient or caregiver depression or anxiety.[91] Talking about end-of-life wishes and fears does not adversely affect the therapeutic alliance[92] and can actually enhance rather than extinguish the patient's sense of hope.[93]

Fear of Illness or Death

One study indicated that medical students may fear death more than other students and that practicing physicians fear death even more than medical students.[94] Thus, physicians are likely to avoid situations that force them to confront their own vulnerability, such as interacting with dying patients.[95]

Fear of Lacking Knowledge
An inability to say "I don't know" weakens therapeutic relationships because patients sense the physician's lack of candor and begin to suspect that honesty is not valued.[96] When facing a diagnosis with which they have little experience, physicians can acknowledge their lack of experience and their plans to learn more. Physicians need to communicate the message "I don't know, but I will not abandon you, and we will work on this together."

Fear of Lacking Communication Skills Training
Discussions about end-of-life issues are difficult for anyone to initiate, including physicians.[46,50] Physician education on communication has improved significantly over the past decade, with increased inclusion of communication skills training across the training spectrum (medical student, resident, fellow).[8] Despite this, physicians still report feeling unprepared and lacking in skills necessary to communicate with patients, families, and other providers regarding end-of-life concerns.[41]

Listening Barriers
Judgment and Evaluation
When physicians focus on evaluating and judging instead of listening to what a patient is trying to say, they are likely to miss important information.[97] The tendency to evaluate and judge others often increases in difficult and emotional situations, which further impedes effective communication at a time when it is most needed.[84] Instead, physicians must endeavor to create a conversation during which both the patient and the physician seek to understand the other party's interpretation of the facts, their emotions, and the ways in which both affect their self-perceived identities.[98]

Assumption and Certainty
When physicians make assumptions about a patient's feelings or jump to conclusions about what a patient is going to say next, they lose opportunities to hear important information. Making assumptions can interfere with the ability to hear new information. For example, if a physician assumes that a patient's descriptions of pain are based on drug-seeking behavior, he or she may fail to carefully assess for pain or prescribe effective dosages of medication (see *UNIPAC 3*). A physician may feel certain that opioids depress respirations and may not comprehend that individually titrated dosages of some opioids are the agents of choice to relieve dyspnea in patients with terminal illness (see *UNIPAC 4*). Other physicians may assume that only certain religious beliefs are correct, and they may be unable to effectively address a patient's spiritual concerns (see *UNIPAC 2*). Physicians may also make assumptions about a patient's feelings or concerns. For example, when a patient responds to a disclosure of serious news with a statement such as "When will this all be over?", the physician may assume the patient is asking about dying, when in fact he or she may be asking about when the hospitalization or chemotherapy will end. When a patient in severe pain states, "this is awful," one should not

assume that the source of suffering is the pain. Rather, the physician should ask the patient to clarify the source of suffering.

Limited Attention Span

Effective listening requires the ability to concentrate. A patient's attention span may be limited because of the effects of a terminal illness. A physician's attention span may be affected by time constraints, which can result in incomplete interviews or lack of attention when patients talk about family or social issues. Mindful practice has been proposed as a methodology to address many listening and other barriers. It involves careful, nonjudgmental attention to physical and mental actions as one performs everyday tasks. Specific techniques can help hone this level of mindfulness, which can, in turn, provide clinicians with unique insights and clarity.[99]

Hearing Loss

Age-related hearing loss is remarkably common, affecting more than 60% of adults older than 75 years. Hearing loss can impair patient-provider communication, particularly related to end-of-life decision making, and is often overlooked. In a recent study, 88% of responding hospice and palliative medicine providers recalled a situation in which hearing loss resulted in physician-patient communication issues, but only 13% of these providers routinely screen for the impairment.[100]

Strategies for Communicating with a Patient with Hearing Loss[100]

Enunciate words clearly.

Speak slowly.

Speak using a low-pitched tone of voice.

Write information.

Reduce extraneous sounds.

Face the patient.

Ensure the patient is wearing hearing aids.

Utilize a pocket talker amplification device.

Avoid shouting, speaking in the patient's ear, and communicating with caregiver only.

Adapted from Hearing Loss in Hospice and Palliative Care: A National Survey of Providers (Table 2), by Smith AK, Ritchie CS, Wallhagen ML, J Pain and Sympt Manage, 2016;52(2):254-258. ©2016 by the American Academy of Hospice and Palliative Medicine. Published by Elsevier, Inc. All rights reserved.

Organizational/System Barriers

Environment and Reimbursement Issues

The current healthcare environment and reimbursement structure discourage adequate physician-patient communication.[60] When patients are grappling with news of a terminal diagnosis, poor prognosis, uncontrolled pain, or painful psychological and spiritual issues, the visit may require more than the usual 15-minute appointment to establish an ongoing relationship with the patient and family. During this visit, it is important to identify psychological, social, and spiritual problems; ensure that patients and family members understand the information being conveyed; and include patients and family members in treatment decisions.

There is evidence that effective communication does not always require a longer visit. In fact, effective communication may shorten patient visits. As little as 40 seconds of compassionate communication can improve perception of the physician and reduce patient anxiety.[101] Visits during which the physician responded to a patient's direct or indirect comments about their emotions were shorter than visits in which the physician ignored these clues.[102]

Standards of Performance

Physicians who are sensitive to the importance of effective communication are more likely to communicate well. They are also more likely to attend workshops to improve their skills, compared with clinicians who need to improve the most.[60] Promoting attendance at appropriate workshops and improving communication performance should be part of an organization's overall risk management strategy and is likely to result in better patient care. Research-based teaching strategies and minimum standards of performance are needed.

Lack of Organizational Support

Encouraging attendance at communication workshops[60] and participation on interdisciplinary teams (IDTs) indicates an organization's support for adequate patient care. Unfortunately, this support is often lacking.[95]

Disparities in Access and Information

Unfortunately many demographic groups in America still lack awareness of and access to quality care for serious illness. Despite receiving less medical care than white patients through most of their lives, non-white patients, particularly African Americans, receive more intense life-prolonging care at the end of life. As such, African American patients are less likely to know about hospice and to enroll.[103] Exposure to information about hospice among this population is associated with more favorable beliefs about what hospice can provide.[104]

Language Barriers

Medical Language

Physicians speak at least two languages: everyday language and medical language. Effective communication depends on the physician's ability to let go of hard-earned medical vocabulary and use words that patients can understand. For example, using the word *shot* may be more effective than *injection, drip* clearer than *infusion,* and *rapid heartbeat* may be more effective than *tachycardia* or *flutter* when communicating common medical vocabulary to patients.

Limited English Proficiency

In the United States, approximately 9% of the population (25 million US residents) meet the definition of limited English proficiency (LEP), meaning they self-identify as speaking English less than "very well." Patients with LEP are at a higher risk of having poor understanding of diagnoses and experiencing miscommunications with their physicians. Physicians can improve communication with patients with LEP by using trained bilingual interpreters. The Selected Communication Issues subsection on Limited English Proficiency on page 90 provides a practical guide for communicating effectively with patients with LEP via medical interpreters.

Vocabulary

Words such as *hospice care, feeding, depression, pain,* and *suffering* are frequently used when caring for someone with a serious illness, but these terms are likely to have different meanings for patients, family members, nurses, physicians, social workers, and chaplains.[105] To improve communication, physicians should choose their words carefully and explain the terms with which patients may be unfamiliar. It is also important to clarify with patients their understanding of terms they are using without making assumptions. For example, an oncologist may describe a patient's cancer as metastatic during patient visits, and the patient may then repeat this to other healthcare providers. While this term means "incurable disease" to healthcare professionals, the patient may not share this same understanding, and continued conversation without a shared understanding of language will lead to communication difficulties. Learning patients' stories and the ways in which they understand their illnesses can help guide language choices.

In most people's minds *eating* refers to the physical act of chewing and swallowing food, and *feeding* refers to spooning food into someone else's mouth. When discussing artificial nutrition, it is better to explain the treatment in nontechnical language and to avoid statements such as "We will continue feeding the patient." The emotional connotations associated with feeding interfere with appropriate cessation of artificial nutrition or hydration when it no longer serves its therapeutic goal (see *UNIPAC 6*).

When using the word *depression,* physicians should distinguish the psychiatric condition of depression from everyday feelings of sadness and grief associated with losses related to terminal illness. Patients may exhibit depressive symptoms such as crying, sadness, and sleep difficulties without meeting the *DSM-5* criteria for depression (see *UNIPAC 2*).

The phrase "nothing can be done" is never helpful, nor is the phrase "withdraw care." The team may decide to "withdraw life support," but they never stop their care of the patient. When curative measures are no longer appropriate, intensive symptom control and an ongoing supportive presence are always possible and appropriate (see *UNIPAC 1*). Choosing phrases that focus on what *can* be done for the patient (symptom management, legacy), rather than what *cannot* be done (dialysis, resuscitation), are more helpful in fostering support and coping.

Patients, family members, and healthcare professionals may mistakenly associate the word *hospice* with loss of hope, lack of medical care, uncontrolled pain, bed-bound status, and imminent death. Instead, hospice and palliative care focuses on expert symptom control; caring support by a team of compassionate, skilled healthcare professionals; strategies to regain and maintain hope; and joyful living until death occurs (see *UNIPAC 1*).

Alternative Approaches to Problematic Phrases

Phrases to Avoid	Phrases to Consider
"Nothing can be done"	"We have reached a point in your care where only treatments that maximize your comfort will be used. Treatments that will not help with comfort will not be continued."
"Withdrawal of care"	"Transition to a care plan focused on providing comfort"

Other Barriers

The lack of privacy in the hospital setting discourages meaningful communication. Televisions and constant interruptions make sustained conversation difficult. In outpatient settings, cold rooms, rigid schedules, and drafty examination gowns inhibit discussion of delicate and troubling issues. Physicians must do their best to overcome these distractions. For example, turning off televisions, shutting hospital room doors, and relocating to a private conference room can be helpful in the hospital. Scheduling extra time for a visit during which tough conversations are expected, allowing patients to dress in their street clothes before initiating conversation, and finding chairs for patients and family members during conversations can be helpful in the outpatient setting.[106]

Strategies for Effective Communication

Quality communication with people with serious illness can be challenging and emotionally charged. As a result, most physicians facing these encounters feel unprepared and uncomfortable with complex communication tasks.[107] A great deal of work demonstrates that patient-centered communication is a learnable skill. Numerous studies show that skills training interventions designed to promote communication skill development are successful in transferring new skills to learners.[8,107-110] In addition, training in relationship-centered communication increases physician empathy and self-efficacy and decreases burnout.[23] To maximize benefit and skills acquisition, communication skills education should include a multimodal approach comprising instruction (lecture, written handouts, modelling), deliberate practice (simulated patient experiences, role-play), and feedback.[8] As with learning any new skill, but especially skills for engaging in end-of-life conversations, learners will be expected to have emotional reactions not only to skill development but also to the content of the conversations. It is important to normalize these challenges and help learners build upon their successes. The remainder of this chapter highlights skills that are fundamental to achieving effective communication and should be considered as part of any communication skills training intervention.

Understand Nonverbal Communication

Much of interpersonal communication is nonverbal; it is conveyed by tone of voice, eye contact, facial expressions, body position, posture, touch, and physical distance.[111] Patients watch physicians for subtle, nonverbal cues communicating the true nature of their condition.[112] When a physician's nonverbal cues contradict their verbal messages, patients are much more likely to believe the nonverbal cues.[113] When physicians smile continually and speak rapidly when delivering serious news, they convey their own discomfort, discourage questions, and confuse the patient. Conversely, nonverbal signals that communicate empathy can be employed to increase comfort and minimize fear and anxiety when discussing difficult topics. A list of useful nonverbal communication skills is found below.

Nonverbal cues are culturally influenced[62] and can be difficult to interpret. Even experts misinterpret nonverbal cues up to 50% of the time.[113] When a patient's nonverbal communication appears to contradict a verbal message, physicians should ask for clarification.[89,115] For example, when patients say they are feeling fine but their eyes are filled with tears, the physician should gently mention the discrepancy, then sit quietly and give the patient a chance to talk about what is really going on. For example, "As we talk, I notice that your eyes are filled with tears. Can you tell me something about what you are feeling?" or "As we talk, I notice that you are looking out the window. Does that mean you are uncomfortable with what we're talking about?"

The meanings assigned to nonverbal communication vary by culture. In general, European cultures view some sustained eye contact as interest. Native American, Asian American, and African American cultures are more likely to view continual eye contact as threatening, hostile, or impolite. When in doubt, it may be helpful to follow the patient's cues.[62]

Nonverbal Communication Skills[114]

Sit at eye level with the patient or slightly lower.

Sit as close to the patient as the relationship dictates.

Sit in a relaxed position with body facing the patient.

Lean toward the patient.

Maintain eye contact.

Use silence to allow patients time with their thoughts.

Use touch as the relationship dictates.

Keep tissues available and within reach of the patient.

Social touch (physical contact in a social context to display caring, such as a hug) can be another form of effective nonverbal communication when employed appropriately. As with other nonverbal cues, the role and acceptability of touch varies greatly by culture and individual; this holds true for both patient and physician. If the use of touch to express caring comes naturally to the physician, patient cues should be followed to determine if touch would be welcomed. Nonverbal body language indicating that the patient is comfortable with touch and finds it reassuring includes leaning toward the physician, continuing to hold the physician's hand when it is offered, and leaning into a hug instead of withdrawing. When a patient's nonverbal communication (drawing back, tensing up, and fidgeting) might indicate discomfort with physical proximity, physicians should move farther away. However, sitting too far away often communicates fear or lack of interest.

Encourage Patients to Talk and Listen to What They Say

Encouraging patients to talk and then listening attentively are critical components of an assessment. As one patient said, "I think it's up to the caregiver, whoever it is, to lead the patient, draw it out of the patient with questions like, 'What are your concerns?' 'What would you like to know?'"[116] In their haste, physicians may not do this; they tend to interrupt patients within the first 18 seconds of an interview and rely on one communication technique—closed questions—that elicit only limited types of information.[117] Allowing patients to voice their full list of concerns at the beginning of an interview can take only 6 seconds longer and result in fewer concerns that may arise later.[118]

Narrative medicine is a particularly helpful construct for hospice and palliative medicine practitioners. This practice focuses on *listening* to the patient's story of her illness, *honoring* its meaning, and *responding* to it. It focuses on empathetic presence and allows the patient and family to self-organize their goals and values within the structure of their narrative. This allows the physician a deeper understanding of the key issues that may influence treatment plans.[44,119] *Dignity therapy* represents one approach to uncovering this narrative. It is a psychotherapeutic intervention that involves questions about the patient's life history, legacy, and accomplishments. It also helps patients define the things they still want to say to their loved ones, including hopes, dreams, advice, and practical instructions. Dignity therapy results in the creation of a document that is shared with the patient's family or friends[120] and has been shown to improve self-reported end-of-life experiences.[121] For more on dignity therapy, see UNIPAC 2.

The communication strategies described in **Table 4** encourage patients to share information about their physical, emotional, social, and spiritual concerns.[97] Listening, acknowledging, clarifying, reassuring, and validating are not just techniques to elicit information; they also serve as powerful therapeutic interventions because they create a healing context and influence the patient's expectations. These interventions also encourage compliance, affect the patient's emotional and physical well-being, and enable patients to describe not only their physical symptoms but also their thoughts, feelings, concerns, fears, frustrations, and expectations.[122]

Ask Before Telling

Before giving any new information, it is generally best to ask the patient or family member about what they already know.[114,123] For example, if you plan to discuss a transition to hospice, it will be a much different conversation with patients who say they do not even know about their terminal diagnosis than it will be with patients who tell you they just spoke to their oncologist (who recommended hospice) and need to know which one serves their area. Some practitioners advocate an "ask-tell-ask" (see **Table 5**) approach for sharing information, in which the clinician asks what the patient knows, tells any new information, and then asks for any questions or concerns.[114,123,124]

Respond with Empathy

Empathy refers to the ability to put aside personal agendas and see the situation from the patient's point of view. An empathetic response communicates the physician's awareness and acceptance of the patient's emotions—not only to listen to a patient's words but to hear the unspoken messages beneath them.[46]

Empathetic relationships are a medium of healing.[122] When physicians respond with empathy, they create an atmosphere in which patients and family members feel free to voice their deepest concerns without fear of rejection, isolation, or abandonment. An empathetic presence helps patients and families relax in the present moment, which is almost always less frightening than worrying about the past or future.

Two of the most pressing challenges associated with empathy are *remaining present* when the patient's suffering evokes the physician's own fears and insecurities and *resisting the almost irresistible need to take action* when listening is more appropriate.[125] The ultimate test of

Table 4. Effective Communication Strategies

Strategies	Examples
Open-Ended Questions Open-ended questions give patients permission to describe their symptoms more fully and to say more about what they are thinking and feeling. Closed questions rarely elicit additional information, but they are appropriate when patients are exhausted, in pain, have cognitive impairment, or when specific information is needed quickly.	"What are some of the things you want to talk about today?" "What is on your mind today?" "Tell me about your pain." "What else can you tell me about where the pain is and how it feels?" "Tell me about your breathing." "Can you tell me more about how you are feeling today?" "Can you tell me something about how your family is coping?"
Minimal Leads and Accurate Verbal Following Minimal leads indicate interest and encourage patients to continue talking. Minimal nonverbal leads include nodding the head, eye contact, and leaning toward the speaker.	**Minimal Leads** "Uh-huh" "Umm" "Hmm" "Ah" **Verbal Following** "Oh?" "Then?" "And?"
Repetition Repetition involves repeating one or two key words from the patient's last sentence to indicate that the physician is listening. This encourages the patient to keep talking and enhances his or her sense of being heard. Repetition does not mean the physician agrees with the patient, but only that the physician is listening. Although repetition is an important skill, it should be mixed with other techniques.	Patient: "When I take the pills I feel nervous." Physician: "The pills make you feel nervous."

Continued on page 23

Table 4. Effective Communication Strategies (continued)

Strategies	Examples
Paraphrasing and Reflecting When physicians paraphrase and reflect, they repeat a patient's statement in their own words to ensure the patient's message is understood.	"Your medication wasn't delivered until 9 pm, then, when you took the pills, they kept you up all night." "When the pain returned, you began to feel anxious and worried." "When you think about dying, you worry about uncontrollable pain."
Clarifying Responses Clarifying responses help physicians understand the facts and the patient's feelings and attitudes. Clarifying responses also help patients think about what they have just said, examine their choices, and look at their life patterns.	"Is it possible that you feel…?" "Can you give me an example of what you are talking about?" "You say you are feeling good most of the time; what is going on when you are not feeling well?" "In the past, how have you coped when sad things happened?" "If you do that, how is it likely to affect your family?"
Confrontation and Honest Labeling This technique gently explores uncomfortable subjects, such as distortions of reality or differences between words and actions. This technique does not necessitate a demand that patients confront their mortality or any other subject.	"When you talk about your wife, you say you understand why she doesn't visit you more often, but I see tears in your eyes. Can you tell me more about how you feel when she doesn't visit?"
Integrating and Summarizing These techniques help to ensure that the patient's main concerns are understood. They help physicians and patients clarify their thoughts and feelings and encourage them to further explore confusing issues.	"Let me see if I understand what you have told me. When the pain returned, you thought it meant you were going to die soon, which made you feel frightened and alone, and you thought about ending your life. However, if the pain can be controlled and people come to visit you, you'd rather live a little longer because you have some important things you'd like to do before you die."

Table 5. Ask-Tell-Ask[114,123,124]

Ask	Assess patient understanding	What have the doctors told you so far?
		To make sure that we're on the same page, can you tell me what is your understanding of your illness?
		What are you expecting the next couple of weeks and months to look like?
Tell	Provide information	Provide small "chunks" of information using straightforward language and avoid jargon. Pause after "chunks" to allow time for processing.
Ask	Check understanding	To make sure my explanation was effective, tell me in your own words what you understand from what I have told you.
		What questions do you have about what we have just discussed?

empathetic presence is being, not doing, captured in the phrase "Don't just do something, sit there!"

Physicians also can show empathy through appropriate physical contact. This involves following the patient's lead regarding physical contact and remembering that holding a hand or giving a hug can have a strong and lasting positive effect if done at the right time with the right patient.[126] Empathetic physicians are sensitive to the inherently unequal nature of the patient-physician relationship, and they do all they can to help patients retain a sense of autonomy and self-worth.

Use of empathetic statements and communication techniques have been shown to improve patient satisfaction with communication.[127] Specific strategies and communication techniques are discussed in more detail in the Communicating Serious News chapter on page 29 (see Respond to the Patients' Feelings). Unfortunately, many opportunities to act with empathy are missed.[128,129] These missed opportunities reflect worries that attending to emotions may open a Pandora's box that will impair a clinician's ability to get through a busy day. One study of oncologists, however, revealed that responding to emotions only lengthened the interview by 21 seconds,[130] and another study showed an empathetic response actually shortened the visit.[102] Attending to emotion can help patients process the news and move on to cognitive information with less anxiety[101] and better recall.[131] Use of other team members often can be helpful, especially for patients with particularly strong emotions, and may lead to better assessment of socioemotional factors.[132]

Manage Uncertainty

Uncertainty is common throughout the disease course for patients with serious illness. For some patients, this uncertainty provides a source of hope; for others, it provides a source of anxiety. Either way, patients grapple with this uncertainty and look to their physician for guidance. Responding in a manner that acknowledges and confronts the uncertainty is necessary to achieve effective patient-centered communication. Although physicians may have a tendency to attempt to minimize uncertainty because of their inherent discomfort in not "having the answer," uncertainty is not a foe. When managed appropriately, uncertainty can provide a structure to cultivate coping.[133]

One helpful strategy for managing uncertainty is to contrast the hope and worry aspects of the situation.[8,133] This can be used to help assess and promote prognostic awareness, which will be discussed in more detail in the section on Gauging Prognostic Awareness (page 57). In addition, statements starting with "I wish…" align patients and physicians through the implicit acknowledgment that the likely outcome will be undesirable or emotionally difficult and that both parties are limited in their control of the outcome. Statements of support and nonabandonment are paramount in situations of high clinical uncertainty and promote a trusting patient-physician relationship.[133] Often patients may be hesitant to address the uncertainty of their situation. Reflective, summative, and empathetic statements can be helpful to promote exploration and normalization of emotions, allowing for resolution of ambivalence and continued discussion.[133] Examples of strategies to manage uncertainty and promote prognostic awareness while expressing empathy and nonabandonment are found in **Table 6** and are revisited in the section on Troubleshooting Prognosis (page 62) and in Tables 16 and 17 (pages 63-64).

Table 6. Strategies to Manage Uncertainty

Assess prognostic awareness	**Hope and worry** Putting together everything that we have talked about, what are you hoping for and what are you worried about?
Promote prognostic awareness	**Hope and worry** I am hopeful that your cancer will respond to this clinical trial. I also worry that your body is so frail that you will not be able to tolerate the therapy. **I wish…** I wish I had more answers for you as to why your body is not responding to the treatment in the way we had hoped. I wish that I could promise you that you will always be there for your daughter.
Nonabandonment	No matter what happens… We will be here…. We will help you…
Reflective statements to normalize emotion	I can see that you have a good understanding of how serious your loved one's situation has become and that you are frightened to think about the future. Do I have this correct?

Use Appropriate Humor

Appropriate humor is a powerful intervention for coping with loss.[134-136] In a large national survey, 93% of seriously ill patients and 87% of bereaved family members said that maintaining a sense of humor was very important.[137] Patients feel that humor between themselves and their care team is appropriate, with those who considered themselves "funny" placing more value on humor during their illness.[138] However, sensitivity and intuition are critical when using humor in palliative care settings.[68]

In his book *Holyquest: The Search for Wholeness,* Anthony Perrino suggests that the nature of true humor lies less in being funny or telling jokes than in kind contemplation of life's incongruities.[140] According to Perrino, true humor has emotional and spiritual significance. It relieves tension, punctures pretense, and restores perspective; allows the mind to function more effectively; and enables people to deal with difficulties more creatively. True humor enhances a sense of wholeness—when people can laugh at themselves, they are reinforcing their identity apart from an event or condition and reflecting on their ability to transcend current circumstances. When used properly, humor enables people to contemplate life's incongruities without anxiety or anger.[140]

Because humor requires perspective, it usually is effective only when people can step back from a situation and recognize its paradoxical qualities. When patients or healthcare providers are suddenly confronted by the deeply tragic aspects of human existence and temporarily engulfed by overwhelming emotions, maintaining a sense of perspective is difficult. During these times, attempts at humor are inappropriate. The recovery process is better served by providing calm, ongoing support as patients and professionals search for a renewed and enlarged sense of meaning and purpose. When some sense of perspective is regained, periodic, gentle humor and lightheartedness with patients and team members may once again be appropriate.

Patients with terminal illnesses have identified several strategies to maintain a sense of hope in the face of their illness, one of which is a lighthearted approach to situations. Patients indicate that healthcare professionals may be the only people with whom they can share humor about their situation. "Humor makes me feel that the person knows I'm still alive; if I can laugh, I feel like I still have some power."[141]

Researchers in the field of *gelotology,* the study of physiological reactions to humorous events, suggest that in most situations physical reactions to humor are beneficial. Laughter reduces stress, aids ventilation, accelerates the exchange of residual air, exercises the myocardium, increases arterial and venous circulation, and reduces vascular stasis.[135]

Characteristics of Therapeutic Humor[139]

Therapeutic humor

- is appropriate and timely
- builds confidence
- brings people together
- recognizes common dilemmas and paradoxes.

Therapeutic humor does not

- ridicule others
- destroy confidence
- diminish teamwork.

Humor as Therapy

The following anecdote illustrates the essence of true humor: appreciating life's paradoxes, accepting human frailties, and integrating the nature of human existence into life without bitterness or sarcasm.

A middle-aged man with a brain tumor was dying in the same manner with which he had lived his life–cantankerously, irascibly, and continually making mountains out of molehills. When the patient's wife and teenage son returned from the hospital cafeteria, they found him sprawled across his bed, exposing himself, and yelling at the staff. The physician was called by a distressed nurse. Instead of focusing on the possible contributing factors to his delirium and its pharmacologic management, the physician sat down with the family. As the patient's wife and son recounted the distressing story, the son looked up and said, "You know, Dad never was willing to go along with the program." Infectious laughter ensued.

By letting go of his need to control the situation and participating in this moment of insight and acceptance of this man's lifelong frailties, the physician helped this mother and son regain a sense of perspective and accept their common dilemma with tolerance, compassion, and humor.

Communicating Serious News

No news is not good news, it is an invitation to fear.[142]

—CM Fletcher

Bad news pertains to "situations where there is either a feeling of no hope, a threat to a person's mental or physical well-being, a risk of upsetting an established lifestyle, where a message is given which conveys to an individual fewer choices in his or her life."[126]

—Robert Bor, et al.

An expert in breaking bad news is not someone who gets it right every time—he or she is merely someone who gets it wrong less often, and who is less flustered when things do not go smoothly.[59]

—Robert Buckman

Communicating serious news is generally regarded as one of the most difficult tasks of medicine. Patients have identified a need for improvement in physician skills in this area.[143] Despite physicians' and families' concerns, studies indicate that patients usually prefer to have information about their diagnosis and prognosis, even when the news is worse than expected.[142] Physicians may fear that communicating the truth will harm patients, but most patients report positive results of being told serious news. Having a label for their condition can explain patients' symptoms and reduce their sense of uncertainty.

When serious news about diagnosis and prognosis is withheld from a patient who wants to know all the details, the patient is more likely to have negative reactions. Learning about a diagnosis by accident or from someone other than the physician in charge can cause distress and confusion. Patients may feel patronized when physicians withhold important information or lonely and isolated when they sense that something is very wrong but cannot talk about it. Many patients also feel it is important that family members do not find out about the diagnosis and prognosis before they do; this can result in a loss of trust in professional and family caregivers.[144] On the other hand, especially in certain cultures, some patients do not want to hear serious news and prefer that physicians talk to their family regarding medical details.

Because judgments about the severity of serious news are subjective, physicians should avoid making assumptions about the ways in which serious news will affect a patient. It is for this reason that many have advocated renaming the act of disclosing information that may seriously or adversely affect a patient's view of the future as "serious," rather than "bad," news. For example, a patient may be relieved to hear a diagnosis of cancer instead of amyotrophic lateral sclerosis.

Serious news is emotionally distressing for recipients, and the manner in which it is communicated is critical. Empathy may be the distinguishing characteristic of clinicians perceived as providing comfort when delivering serious news compared with those whose manner causes further distress. The only tolerable aspect of hearing serious news often is the physician's deep concern and empathy with the patient's plight. **Table 7** describes patients' preferences when physicians share distressing news.[142]

Hospice and palliative care physicians rarely need to communicate the initial serious news about a terminal diagnosis. More often, they communicate serious news about the meaning of changes in the patient's condition, such as when a patient has entered the terminal phase of what may have been a chronic illness. For example, patients with serious, chronic diseases such as breast cancer, prostate cancer, congestive heart failure, HIV/AIDS, or emphysema may cope with their diagnosis fairly well for several years and then suddenly need to face the full implications of their condition.[145,146] The following guidelines are applicable in all settings of serious news, from the initial disclosure to any major changes throughout the illness experience.

General Guidelines for Communicating Serious News

Disclosing information should not be a one-time event; instead, communication should be an ongoing process, with the pace of disclosure determined by the patient's personality, coping mechanisms, and desire to know more.[68]

Studies indicate that physicians, nurses, and other team members consistently underestimate the amount of information patients want and misinterpret the kinds of information they desire.[68] Physicians often want to talk about diagnosis and treatment, but patients more often want information about the disease's likely impact on their lives and their family members, how their prognosis is likely to affect their future plans, psychological issues related to their diagnosis and prognosis, and available resources to cope with daily living.[68]

Most patients with a terminal illness know they are dying; avoiding discussions of prognosis is likely to increase their sense of loneliness and abandonment and deny them opportunities for meaningful communication about death-related issues. Some patients may prefer ambiguous information that allows them to continue hoping for a cure, but in most cases lack of information only increases stress and anxiety, particularly when patients suspect the true diagnosis.[68]

Table 7. Patients' Preferences When Physicians Communicate Serious News

Direct, empathetic communication

Information about the diagnosis that provides a label for their condition

Information about the prognosis and ways the illness is likely to affect their quality of life

Inclusion of a family member or trusted friend in the discussion

Encouragement to ask questions

Information that is neither overly optimistic nor overly pessimistic

Practical information about what to do and how to obtain additional information

Many factors contribute to the experience of receiving serious news. A personalized approach to delivering serious news requires consideration of patient's individual needs (preferences for information and handling of emotions), family relationships, systemic and institutional factors, and cultural environment.[147] When receiving serious news, patients value recognition of their experience hearing the news and guidance toward what should be done next. Patients also find it important for clinicians to be responsive to their fluctuating needs for recognition and guidance and to be able to move back and forth between them as necessary.[148]

Clinical Situation

Juanita

You are a physician working in an outpatient palliative care clinic located in a multidisciplinary group practice (primary care, palliative care, oncology, etc.). During your clinic, a primary care physician (PCP) walks into your office and asks for your help with one of her patients. The patient, Juanita, is a 65-year-old woman with a recent history of vague abdominal pain and weight loss. The workup for these symptoms revealed a large pancreatic mass that was possibly cancerous; biopsy confirms this concern. The patient is returning today to discuss the test results. The PCP has a long-standing relationship with this patient and feels "distraught" at the thought of having to tell Juanita this "terrible" news, especially since Juanita can be "extremely emotional." Because you are good in "really tough" situations, the PCP asks for your help delivering this serious news. In preparation for this meeting, the PCP encouraged Juanita to bring a supportive family member. Juanita has brought her husband, Al, whom the PCP has never met.

- What communication techniques can you use to encourage patients to share information about their physical, emotional, social, and spiritual concerns?

- Why is it important to address emotions, and what are some nonverbal ways you can respond to an emotional patient?

- How will you know if a patient would respond positively to touch?

- How can you determine how much the patient wants to know?

Case continues on page 43

A Six-Step Protocol for Communicating Serious News

Several protocols for communicating serious news are available.[16,46,52,149-151] Each of these protocols, at their core, comprise similar components and communication tasks. Compassion and a caring human presence are always essential components of communicating serious news. In addition, the following six steps have improved communication in many difficult circumstances:

1. Arrange the physical context and the emotional atmosphere.
2. Find out how much the patient knows.
3. Find out how much the patient wants to know.
4. Share information (align and educate).
5. Respond to the patient's feelings.
6. Make a plan and follow through.

The SPIKES protocol[152] (**Table 8**) is one example of a commonly taught and employed protocol for delivering serious news. SPIKES serves as a helpful mnemonic to guide physicians through complex communication encounters using six steps.[152]

Arrange the Physical Context and the Emotional Atmosphere

Planning takes a few minutes, but it saves time and distress in the long run, particularly when serious news must be shared and the patient's reactions are likely to be emotional.

Before the interview, review the medical facts of the case, any major concerns previously voiced by the patient or family, and relevant family dynamics. Arrange for unhurried, uninterrupted time in a private room or at the patient's home, where patients and family members can ask questions and express themselves freely. Turn pagers to a silent setting and reroute telephone calls if possible.

Negotiate who should deliver the information. This person is usually the doctor, but some patients might want information delivered by others, such as a clergy or family member. Negotiate who should be present during the discussion.[153] Involvement of a trusted primary care physician (PCP) is often helpful and has been associated with higher satisfaction.[154] If the patient agrees, include a family member or friend in the interview so the patient feels less alone and has someone to talk with after the physician leaves. A friend or family member also can help provide support for the patient and serve as a witness to what was said and how the news was delivered. The presence of a friend or family member also gives the physician an opportunity to model open and compassionate communication about death and dying, which can help prepare friends and family members for the patient's death. Elderly patients in particular prefer to have family present,[155] and having someone there has been associated with improved recall of things that were said.[131] If no family member or friend is available, including a nurse or other team member in the interview is helpful for many of the same reasons. The presence of a trained nurse during disclosure of serious news has been associated with lower distress and better long-term coping.[156]

Table 8. SPIKES Protocol for Communicating Serious News[152]

Step	Context	Description/Suggested Phrases
Setting	Prepare before the meeting.	Review pertinent medical facts (chart review and discussion with consultants).
		Provide a quiet, private location.
		Ensure that key stakeholders are present.
		Ensure that tissues are available.
		Ensure sufficient seating for all participants.
		Minimize distractions (silence phones/pagers).
Perception	Assess how the patient views the medical situation.	"What is your understanding of what is going on?"
		"What have the other doctors told you about your health?"
Invitation	Ask permission to talk about a sensitive topic.	"Would it be okay if we talked about the results of your scan?"
		"Would it be ok with you if we discussed something that has been worrying me?"
Knowledge	Provide the medical facts.	Give a warning.
		"I have something serious we need to discuss."
		Use concise, simple language without technical/medical jargon.
		Allow time for questions and processing.
Empathy	Attend to patient emotions.	Therapeutic silence
		NURSE Statements (see Table 10, page 39)
		"I know this is not what you expected to hear today."
		"This is very difficult news."
Summary	Discuss next steps and a follow-up plan.	"So I know that I explained myself clearly, could you summarize what we just talked about?"
		"What are you planning on telling your family when they ask about this meeting?"

Arrange the environment so physical barriers such as bedside tables and trays do not interfere with verbal and nonverbal communication. Televisions and radios should be turned off. Arrange seating in a way that encourages communication; the physician should sit close enough to the patient to attend to his or her emotional responses and provide therapeutic touch when needed and appropriate. A distance of 2 to 3 feet is usually comfortable during personal discussions, but follow the patient's cues; some patients may need more or less personal space. If possible, place the physician's chair at a right angle to the patient instead of behind a desk or across the room.[115] Make sure facial tissues are within everyone's reach.

When delivering serious news, it is vital to establish a caring relationship. Before speaking, make introductions to acknowledge the presence of all parties and determine their relationships. Introduce everyone in the room, including other healthcare professionals. Shaking hands is a matter of cultural and personal preference. If cultural norms support handshaking, shake the patient's hand first if possible, even when other family members are present.

The most important rule when delivering serious news to a patient is to sit down, even when chairs must be brought from another room. In one study, despite saying identical words, physicians who sat for the discussion were rated as more compassionate.[157]

Find Out How Much the Patient Knows

Before communicating serious news, find out what information has already been shared with the patient, the patient's impression of the seriousness of the illness, how the illness is currently affecting the patient's daily life, and the patient's understanding of the likely prognosis. Answers to these questions can help physicians decide which information to share first and how to share it. After asking a question, stop and give the patient sufficient time to answer. This is the first "ask" in the ask-tell-ask approach previously described.

Patients may say that other physicians have told them nothing about their illness, but anxiety often interferes with a patient's ability to hear and retain information. Patients may also be hoping to hear different information this time and therefore may not want to bias the physician by sharing prior difficult news. Alternatively, patients may have developed their own narrative or understanding of their illness that often makes it difficult to hear medical facts. Attempting to understand this narrative will give valuable guidance on how to discuss the medical facts in a way that is more acceptable to patients. Confronting patients or expressing amazement or concern about their lack of knowledge or the communication habits of other physicians is not helpful. Asking the patient to describe their illness experience in their own words can help identify hidden stories, emotions, or questions and can be a helpful approach in this scenario. Although often effective, the question "What is your understanding of your disease?" occasionally can be perceived as a test of knowledge and cause patients and families to feel defensive. Examples of other open-ended questions are found in **Table 9**.

Table 9. Statements for Eliciting Patient Perspective[46]

Assess the patient's cognitive perspective on the illness.

"What is your understanding of the situation you and your family are facing right now?"

"What has the doctor told you about your illness?"

"What did your doctor tell you when you were referred for hospice and palliative care? What does that mean to you?"

"How serious does your illness seem to be?"

"Did you think something serious was going on when…?"

"What are your expectations from your illness? For the future?"

Assess the patient's emotional perspective on the illness.

"Tell me more about how you are feeling about your illness."

"Tell me more about how you are making sense of all of this."

"Tell me more how your illness is impacting your life."

Find Out How Much the Patient Wants to Know

Discovering how much patients want to know is an important part of the communication process.[153] Although patients have a right to full disclosure of truthful information and usually desire it, some do not. Unfortunately, there is no way to predict how much disclosure is desired, and the only way to know is to gently ask patients how much they want to know and remind them they can end the interview whenever they need to and delegate the sharing of information to family members or others. A follow-up interview can be scheduled after they have had a chance to assimilate the news.

Be sensitive to the patient's needs, and consider questions such as the following:

- "Sometimes people want to know all the details about their condition, sometimes they just want to know the big picture, and sometimes they don't want to know anything and prefer I talk to a family member. What do you want?"
- "What is the most important information for you to have now?"
- "Do you want to hear the basic facts now and then talk more at a later time?"
- "Do you want to hear information directly or through a family member?"
- "Please let me know if you feel that I am sharing too much information."

Share Information (Align and Educate)

Physicians often underestimate a patient's desire for knowledge and may spend little more than 1 minute of a 20-minute interview sharing information.[158] On the other hand, too much emphasis on dispensing knowledge, often at the expense of assessing patient perspective or attending to emotion, can be equally detrimental. Effective communication takes time and a patient-centered approach. It requires tailoring information to the patient's needs, determining his or her understanding of what has been said, and clarifying misunderstandings.

Use Plain Language

When sharing serious news with a patient, promise to answer questions openly and honestly. Choose vocabulary carefully and use simple, everyday language (eg, no medical jargon, euphemisms, or technical or diagnostic terminology). Use the patient's factual understanding and style of communication to guide information sharing. When medical terminology is required or requested by patients or families, first explain the medical terms in plain language.

Encourage patients and family members to take notes. Some physicians suggest that patients record conversations so they can refer to the tape later; however, medical or legal concerns may present challenges to recording conversations.

Adapt to the Patient's Communication Style

Use the same general vocabulary as the patient. Use caution when communicating with patients who use medical language; their understanding of the terminology may be faulty. It is helpful to ask patients to explain in their own words what that terms means to them. Remain cautious when communicating with patients who are healthcare professionals; their emotional responses are like those of any other patient, and they are likely to experience similar difficulties hearing and retaining distressing information.

Fire "Warning Shots" When Needed

When large gaps exist between the patient's knowledge and medical reality, verbal messages should indicate that the situation is more serious than the patient realizes.

💡 Warning Shots

I have some news that may be difficult to hear.

I'm afraid the situation is more serious than we thought.

Share Information in Small Steps

After the "warning shot" is delivered, it is best to share the serious news clearly and succinctly in one or two sentences. It is important to avoid euphemisms that may be misunderstood and to define any unclear terms. Examples of short, clear statements include
- "Scans show that your cancer is back."
- "The biopsy indicates that you have cancer."
- "Surgery is not going to be possible to repair your valve."

Terms such as "tumor," "mass," and "neoplasm" may be misunderstood. After the news has been shared, it is best to wait quietly for the patient to respond. Often it is not possible to absorb more than the serious news, and further statements are either not heard or allow the patient to "forget" the serious news.

When patients indicate they do not want to hear further information, either directly or indirectly, it is helpful to provide information gradually. This allows patients to determine the pace at which the news is being delivered and is appreciated by most patients as a sensitive approach to the delivery of serious news. A more direct approach is acceptable to some patients if they hold a long-standing relationship with the physician.[159] As the patient's understanding gradually reflects medical reality, remember that stress interferes with the ability to hear and retain information. Physicians may need to repeat information several times during the interview and during the next several days, weeks, or months. Let the patient's reactions dictate how much they are told.

Stop Frequently
When sharing information, stop frequently to assess the following:
- The patient's understanding of what has been said and any misinformation that needs to be corrected. For example, "This must be very confusing. What can I clarify? Can you tell me what you understand so far so I'll know what to talk about next?"
- The patient's emotional response to what has been said. Notice body language and ask patients about their responses to the news. Try not to make assumptions about how the news is affecting them. For example, "Can you tell me something about how this information is affecting you?"
- Unspoken concerns that have not yet been addressed. Ask patients and family members if they have questions that have not yet been answered, then pause long enough to let them formulate questions. For example, "This must be very difficult for you. What are some of the questions or concerns we haven't addressed yet?"
- The patient's ability to continue listening. After hearing the word cancer, patients may not hear another word. Leaving space for silence, acknowledging emotion, and asking a question such as "What are you thinking now?" may help the patient to process the emotion and be receptive to more information. However, at times the patient will not be able to absorb more information. When patients are no longer listening, stop and schedule another interview. Continued attempts to communicate will be unproductive. For example, "This must be very confusing and overwhelming. Do you want to spend some time thinking about what we've discussed so far and then get back together later?"

Provide Information that Patients Want to Know
Physicians and patients often have different goals when sharing information. Physicians tend to emphasize medical information about the disease, such as its stages and possible treatments. Patients often want this information, but they also want information about prognosis and how the symptoms will affect their everyday lives; they want to know how long they will live and how much pain they will have.[57] Try to elicit as many of the patient's concerns as possible.

Provide Information About Prognosis
Patients generally want to know their prognosis[160] and have legitimate needs for the information. Knowing their prognosis allows patients to prioritize their plans for the future[161] and make medical decisions. This can be especially important after receiving serious news that will impact and alter many aspects of a patient's life. The Communicating Prognosis chapter on page 57 provides further discussion on how to approach this discussion.

Respond to the Patient's Feelings
Express Empathy
Emotion is commonly experienced in hospice and palliative care communication encounters. Frequently experienced patient emotions include anxiety, sadness, and anger.[162] Empathy is a key element in any physician-patient interaction. When giving serious news, empathy is especially critical and should be present throughout the interaction.

On average, patients forget about 40% to 80% of the medical information provided by physicians. Emotion evoked by delivery of serious news has been linked to poor information recall during medical encounters.[163] Addressing emotion can be an effective way to help patients manage their emotions and improve recall.

Eliciting, acknowledging, and validating a patient's feelings about diagnosis and prognosis are important aspects of effective communication.[48] Because physicians tend to underestimate a patient's distress,[164,165] deliberate attention to and exploration of patient emotions are essential.[149] Physicians should resist the urge to reassure or fix prematurely, and they need to find ways to sit with the patient and the emotion. Verbal methods to address emotion can be summarized by the mnemonic NURSE (**Table 10**).[129,166]

Another mnemonic for demonstrating empathy that is useful in clinical practice and teaching is SAVE (**Table 11**)[167].

Patients may respond to serious news with stunned silence, anger, disbelief, acute distress, intellectualization, or guilt.[168] When intense distress occurs, physicians sometimes fear the patient's emotions will remain uncontrollable. In most cases, the best response is to wait quietly until emotions subside, generally within a few minutes, followed by a statement of empathy.

When patients begin to cry, try to not distract them by immediately patting them, handing them a tissue, or otherwise interfering. Stay calm, let them experience their emotions, and wait until their body language indicates they are ready for a tissue or a touch. Patients value physicians who acknowledge the patient's emotional response to serious news without becoming emotionally overwhelmed.[148]

When patients respond with anger, let them speak without responding defensively or trying to correct misconceptions. Anger can be the result of displaced fear or feelings of being ignored or devalued. In addition, anger can be a mechanism for tension release or coping.[169] When emotions subside, suggest approaches for the problems that can be fixed. When problems cannot be fixed (eg, death is inevitable), provide reassurance that the patient will not be

Table 10. NURSE Mnemonic: Ways to Verbally Address Emotions[129,166]

Skill	Sample Phrase
Name	I can see that this is frustrating.
	It seems that this is very upsetting to you.
	I wonder if you might be feeling angry.
Understand	I can't imagine how hard this is for you.
	I can only imagine what it is like to balance your treatments with your family life.
	I can't possibly understand what you are going through right now.
	I think I'm understanding you to say that you are concerned about the effect of the chemotherapy on your kids.
Respect	You're doing all the right things and asking the right questions.
	I've been so impressed by the care you have been providing for your wife during the many years of her illness.
Support	I'm going to walk this road with you.
	You're not alone in this.
Explore	Tell me more about what worries you.
	I sense how upset you are feeling about the results of the CT scan.

Table 11. SAVE

Skill	Sample Phrase
Support	Let's work together.
Acknowledge	This has been hard on you.
Validate	Most people would feel the way you do.
Emotion naming	You seem sad.

From "The REDE model of healthcare communication: Optimizing relationship as a therapeutic agent" (Figure 1), by Windover, AK, Boissy A, Rice TW, Merlino J, Gilligan T, & Velez V, J Patient Exper. 2014;1(1):8-13. ©2014 SAGE Publications, Inc. Reprinted by permission of SAGE Publications, Inc.

abandoned, the physician will concentrate on alleviating symptoms, and the entire team will continue providing support and a caring presence.

I wish statements can be particularly powerful when discussing serious news. For example, if the patient says, "There must be something else you can do," the physician can respond, "I wish we had better treatments for your cancer." This conveys the reality of the situation without conveying false hope. It also aligns the physician with the patient and expresses empathy.[170] *We* statements can also be useful. For example, instead of saying, "I know this isn't the result *you* were hoping for," a physician can say, "I know this isn't the result *we* were hoping for." This aligns the patient and physician as members of the same team with common goals.

There are times when empathy alone may not be effective. Consider the above example of the patient's statement "There must be something else you can do." Although this statement often is an emotional response to the realization that time is limited, it also may be a true request for factual information or to continue searching for heroics. Occasionally empathy begets escalating emotion. In these scenarios, empathetic statements are likely to meet resistance (eg, continued requests for facts, frustration). If empathy is attempted and not leading to expected outcomes (ie, raising instead of lowering the emotional temperature), an alternative strategy should be employed that focuses away from NURSE/SAVE statements and back toward the rational and planning mind using Ask-Tell-Ask.[171] **Table 12** summarizes different strategies discussed above to display empathy with patients and families.

Use Appropriate Self-Disclosure
When used appropriately, self-disclosure can be an effective communication tool if the patient's concerns, not the physician's emotional needs, remain the primary focus. Effective self-disclosure depends on the depth of the physician-patient relationship. During a first interview, appropriate self-disclosure may be limited to acknowledging having lived in the same town or sharing a similar hobby. As the relationship continues, physicians can respond to cues indicating that the patient wants a deeper, more human encounter, if professional boundaries are maintained. The following examples illustrate appropriate self-disclosure.

Acknowledging the physician's feelings. After several weeks of home visits from her physician, an elderly hospice patient commented on the physician's tie, saying it was much more conservative than usual. She guessed he would be attending a meeting. The physician complimented her astute observation and acknowledged that he was on his way to a business meeting. When the patient noted that the physician's tone of voice indicated that he was not looking forward to the meeting, the physician laughed and agreed. These few comments established a more personal connection between the patient and her physician while maintaining appropriate professional boundaries (eg, the physician did not go on to complain about the grave differences of opinion he was having with a managed care organization).

Acknowledging shared feelings. When a patient's sister commented on the extreme anger she was experiencing as a result of her brother's terminal illness, the physician responded, "When my brother died, I was angry too. How is the anger affecting you and your relationships with your family?" The physician's response aligned the physician with the sister and acknowledged the validity of her feelings, then redirected the focus of the conversation back to her.

Table 12. Strategies to Display Empathy

Nonverbal Strategies	Therapeutic silence
	Touch (as the relationship dictates)
Empathetic Statements	
NURSE Statements	See Table 10.
SAVE Statements	See Table 11.
I wish…	I wish we had better treatments for your cancer.
	I wish I had more answers for you as to why your body is not responding to treatments as we had hoped.
We (instead of "I")	"I know this isn't the result we were hoping for" (instead of "I know this isn't the result you were hoping for.").

Use Therapeutic Silence

Therapeutic silence is an important part of effective communication. When patients suddenly become quiet, they may be experiencing emotions so strong that they are unable to speak. Physicians should stop, remain quiet for a moment, and then ask about what the patient is thinking and feeling. Until emotional needs are assessed and attended to, patients will be unable to hear further information.

Therapeutic silence allows patients and family members to
- think about what has been said
- assimilate information
- identify and experience feelings
- integrate their intellectual knowledge and emotional needs
- formulate and ask questions.

💡 Transition Statements After a Period of Therapeutic Silence

This must be difficult to hear. Can you tell me something about what you are thinking and feeling?

That was a lot of information. Is it alright if I ask what is going through your mind right now?

Provide Support and Hope
Avoid meaningless statements such as "Everything is going to be fine." Use empathetic statements to provide support without providing false reassurance. Statements such as "We will work on this together" and "We will do everything we can to control your pain, nausea, and breathlessness" convey support and hope. Other statements could include "If we run into problems, we will call on other consultants for help" and "We will do everything we can to make sure you can stay at home."

Understand that a patient's focus of hope is likely to change during the course of an illness and often increases with effective palliative care.[141] Early in the course of a life-threatening illness, the patient's hope may be for a cure, and this may be appropriate. In this scenario, a "hope for the best and prepare for the worst" approach may be effective. This enables patients to retain hope, but it simultaneously prepares them for what most likely lies ahead.[172] Later in the illness, the physician is responsible for helping the patient reframe hope for realistic goals (see *UNIPAC 2*).

Stress nonabandonment at all times. Hearing that there is nothing more the physician can do has been associated with a high level of emotional distress and a perception of the need to improve communication.[143] This statement implies the physician will abandon the patient. A reassurance that the physician will stay with the patient through this process can be invaluable.[32]

Before the interview ends, explain to the patient and family the process they should follow to contact the physician or person on call when they need more information or want to talk. Provide a business card and share telephone numbers. This is particularly important when the interview closes prematurely or when patients are unwilling to discuss important issues.

Make a Plan
Most patients and families want their physicians to help them make sense of the diagnosis and prognosis and provide guidance when making decisions. The Achieving a Shared Decision section on page 53 provides details on how to involve patients and families in the problem-solving process to reinforce their sense of control and competence while achieving a care plan that is mutually appropriate for both patient and physician.

Summarize the Interview
Summarize the interview verbally and in writing, if possible. Ask patients and families to voice their remaining questions, and suggest they keep a list of questions for the next interview.

Make a Contract and Follow Through
Making a contract can be as simple as saying, "I will see you in a week or two." In the home care setting, the contract may be the statement, "The home care team will be visiting you frequently. Let them know about any problems you are experiencing and tell them about any other concerns you may have. Call the hospice and palliative care program if you have questions, and I will get back to you as soon as I can." Be sure to follow through with promises to return calls promptly.

Clinical Situation

Juanita's Case Continues (continued from page 31)

You are the palliative care physician joining the PCP in a meeting with Juanita and her husband, Al. The goal of the meeting is to share test results, which identify that Juanita has pancreatic cancer.

The Conversation	Specific Strategies and Skills
In preparation for the meeting, you and the PCP review the medical facts and negotiate roles. The PCP will start the conversation and look to you when she would like you to take over. Juanita and her husband are in a private consultation room. There are enough chairs for everyone. You enter the room.	Arrange the physical context and the emotional atmosphere
PCP: Hello, Juanita. *(They hug.)* It's good to see you today. Can you introduce me to your family?	
Juanita: This is my husband, Al.	
PCP: Very nice to meet you, Al. I'm grateful to see that Juanita has someone here for support today. I would like to introduce you to my colleague, Dr. Smith, a palliative care physician who works with me here in this office…	
Juanita *(interrupting)*: Well, now I'm really scared. Palliative care—that means you have some terrible news about the test results.	
Juanita looks to the floor and her eyes begin to tear up. The PCP looks to you for help.	Respond to the patient's feelings (**N**URSE [Name]).
You: Juanita and Al, it is very nice to meet you, and thank you for letting me join you today. Juanita, I can see that you are worried about why we are meeting today. Can you tell me what you are worried about?	Respond to the patient's feelings (NURS**E** [Explore]) and find out how much the patient knows.
Juanita raises her eyes from the floor and looks you in the eyes.	

Communication and Teamwork | 43

Juanita: I'm freaking out, actually. I've been worrying about this weight loss for some time now. They keep sending me for more tests. Then, I'm told to bring my husband to talk about the results, which can only mean it's bad news. Now the palliative care doctor is here. *(She pauses.)* I know all about palliative care. My friend with breast cancer saw a palliative care doctor. *(She pauses)* So this means I have cancer?

You: That's a very scary thing to be worried about. It appears to me you are very worried about what we are here to discuss today. At some point, I would like to tell you more about palliative care, but it seems to me you are ready to discuss the results of your tests. Do I have this correct?

Respond to the patient's feelings (**N**URSE [Name]).

Respond to the patient's feelings (N**U**RSE [Understand]).

Find out how much the patient wants to know.

Juanita *(tearfully)*: Yes. I just need to know.

Juanita reaches for Al's hand.

You: Juanita, we have some difficult news to discuss today. *(Pause.)* Your test results show that you have cancer—cancer of the pancreas. *(Allow a period of silence to let Juanita and Al absorb the news.)*

Share information (warning shot).

Share information (clear statement in 1 or 2 sentences followed by silence).

Respond to the patient's feelings (therapeutic silence).

You: This must be difficult to hear. Can you tell me something about what you are thinking and feeling?

Make a transition statement after a period of therapeutic silence.

Juanita is crying. Al's eyes tear up.

Juanita: Cancer. That's what I was afraid of.

You: This isn't the news we were hoping for. Would it be helpful for me to continue, or do you need time to think about this?

Respond to the patient's feelings (*We* statement).

Find out how much the patient wants to know.

Juanita: Time. I need some time to wrap my head around this. Is that okay?

You: Of course. I can only imagine how overwhelming and frightening this must be for you.

Respond to the patient's feelings (N**U**RSE [Understand]).

Although hearing that you have cancer is always life changing, I want you to know that we are here to help you and that we can explore options for treating this cancer. Now that we know what this is, we can get a handle on what to do for you next.	Provide support and hope.
Let's take a break now to give you and your husband time to think about what we have discussed today. Write down any questions you may have. Dr. Smith will call you tomorrow to answer your questions and talk more about next steps. In the meantime, please call sooner if there is something you want to discuss. Does that sound okay?	Make a plan.
Juanita: Yes. That sounds good.	
You: Juanita, can you summarize for me what we discussed today?	
Juanita: Yes. I have cancer. I need some time to figure out what this means. Dr. Smith will call me tomorrow.	Make a plan (summarize the interview and make a contract).
You: That is correct. I look forward to seeing you in a couple days. Please call me if you have any concerns before then.	Make a plan (make a contract). Respond to the patient's feelings (NUR**S**E [Support]).

Case continues on page 50

Special Considerations
Death Notification
In hospice and palliative care, many deaths are "expected" after long experiences with chronic illness or cancer; it is not uncommon for hospice and palliative medicine physicians also to be involved in "unexpected" deaths after trauma, stroke, or other unanticipated events. Regardless of the nature of death, the death of a loved one is a devastating event; bereaved family members will remember the events of the day many years after they occur. The actual act of notifying loved ones of the death itself is especially important because the words and attitudes used by healthcare professionals can greatly impact loved ones during their bereavement.[173]

Death notification is at its core "serious news," and the act of disclosing the death of loved ones is similar to disclosing serious news in other scenarios. The six-step protocol for disclosing serious news described earlier is applicable here with a few additional adaptations and considerations.

Notification should be made as soon as possible. In-person notification is best; avoid telephone notification if possible. Briefly eliciting family members' understanding of events that led up to the death can be helpful in the event a physician does not have a prior relationship with the patient and family (for example, in the event of sudden death from trauma). This will help set the context for delivery of information and subsequent emotional response. When death is expected, as in the case of an actively dying hospice patient, eliciting family members' understanding of the events leading up to the death may not be necessary. When delivering the news, provide a warning shot to alert family members that they are about to hear news that will be difficult. Clearly explain that the patient has died, using the words "death" and "died" and avoiding euphemisms. Family members may wish to hear a detailed explanation of events that led up to the death. After responding to the emotional reaction to the news, share details consistent with the family's desire for information. Expect a strong emotional reaction to the news; respond to this emotion using the strategies described above. Provide contact information for the healthcare team so that the family may obtain answers to questions about the death that may arise later, information on funeral and burial, and local bereavement resources. Have members of the interdisciplinary team present during the discussion if possible, and follow up with family immediately after the notification. Allow family to view and stay with the deceased.

Although it is not preferred because of the impersonal nature and lack of available support, occasionally there are situations that necessitate death notification via telephone. In certain situations, it may be reasonable to request an in-person meeting with the family, requesting their presence to discuss serious news before delivering the death notification. In the event family asks directly about the death of their loved one, honesty is best. When death notification must occur via telephone, there are some strategies that can help improve the communication exchange. While much of the encounter can follow the recommendations above for similar in-person disclosures of serious news, a few additional tips should be considered. Proper introductions to identify the speaker's role and relationship to the family's loved one are important, especially if the speaker is unfamiliar with the family. Inquire about the family member's location. If the family member is driving, request that the family member call back after they reach a safe location. Ask the family member to move to a private location without distractions. It can also be helpful to determine if the family member is alone or has support nearby. Much like delivering serious new in person, a "warning shot" can be helpful. This can be simple and practical, such as, "Are you able to hear some difficult news now?" or "Is now an okay time for me to tell you some difficult news?" Non-verbal demonstrations of empathy are not possible over the phone; therefore, therapeutic silence and empathetic statements are important.[174]

Death notification is difficult for the healthcare team providing the notification, as well. Debriefing after the event can help process the events and the healthcare team members' emotions.[173]

Autopsy

Most physicians feel uncomfortable and unprepared approaching a patient's family to offer them the option of autopsy.[175] There is some evidence that hospice physicians feel that requesting autopsy may be inappropriate. However, many hospital forms and state death certificates require that the physician offer the family the opportunity for autopsy. Consent for autopsy legally must be obtained from the next of kin. It is not sufficient to obtain consent from the patient while he is alive, although conversations with the patient and family may help the family in making this decision. When death is expected, families are often comfortable discussing the option of autopsy when they discuss plans for burial and funeral arrangements. Raising the option before the patient's death allows for family discussion and contemplation but must be done with sensitivity and awareness of the family's comfort with this topic. Autopsy can be beneficial to families if there is a desire to understand the cause of death, give back to society, contribute to medical knowledge, or learn about familial diseases. The next of kin can specify limits to the autopsy (certain organs) and bodies can be viewed after autopsy. The College of American Pathologists published a document on requesting permission for an autopsy. It can be found at http://www.cap.org/apps/docs/committees/autopsy/requesting_consent.doc (Accessed April 24, 2017). When death occurs in the hospital, the hospital assumes the cost for the autopsy; however, when a patient dies at home or outside of the hospital, the family is required to pay for the autopsy and for transporting the patient to the hospital, which can cost anywhere from $500 to $3,000,[17] limiting the practical availability of autopsy for patients who die at home.

Communicating to Achieve a Shared Decision

The concept of shared decision making has its roots in the ethics of consenting for medical treatments such that patients have a right to fully understand and participate in their medical care. According to the Institute of Medicine, shared decision making is the process of communication, deliberation, and decision making during which[11]

- one or more clinicians share with the patient information about relevant testing or treatment options, including the severity and probability of potential harms and benefits and alternatives of these options given the specific nature of the patient's situation
- the patient explores and shares with the clinician(s) his or her preferences regarding these harms, benefits, and potential outcomes
- through an interactive process of reflection and discussion, the clinician(s) and patient reach a mutual decision about the subsequent treatment or testing plan.

As noted earlier, shared decision making is considered the pinnacle of patient-centered communication and is the standard for quality patient care. Achieving a shared decision in practice is not easy, and there remains a gap between the patient's desire for engagement and actual practice.[11] A growing body of literature supports decision aides (tools intended to provide detailed, balanced, evidence-based information about competing treatment options) to facilitate shared decision making in practice.[11] Now more than ever, patients prefer to be active participants in their own medical care and, specifically, to be involved in medical decisions.[11]

Clinical Decisions

For a small number of treatment decisions, there is such unquestionable evidence of benefit with so few downsides that physicians and patients are almost always undivided on the appropriate course of action. Take, for example, the decision to fix a displaced fracture in a child. In such a scenario, where the "right" is so apparent, the role of shared decision making is minimal. At the end-of-life, however, "right" is harder to find. Consider now a fracture in a patient who is bed bound and in hospice with severe dementia who is no longer taking food or liquids. Here the importance of shared decision making is paramount because the benefits and burdens of intervention become less clear and patient (or family) preference becomes much more important.

Eliciting Patient-Specific Goals for Medical Care

Shared decision making is not possible without identifying that which is important to the patient and family. Physicians can help patients and families identify goals for medical care through discussion of patient-specific hopes, concerns, values, and preferences.

There are many possible goals of health care: preventing illness, curing disease, prolonging life, relieving suffering, and improving quality of life, to name a few. No one goal is more valid than any of the others, and multiple goals may apply simultaneously. Each patient and family has personal hopes and goals for their lives—dynamic goals that change as illness shifts—and are influenced by many factors, including past experiences and belief systems. The physician's goal is to help the patient and family consider their medical options in the context of their values and goals.[177] Four questions should be considered when helping patients and families identify goals for medical care[178]:

- Whose goals are being considered?
- Are the goals achievable?
- Are the goals beneficial to the patient?
- How are results measured?

The primary goal setter should be the patient or an appropriate surrogate in the event the patient lacks decision-making capacity. Patients and family members may have conflicting goals. A patient may be exhausted by terminal illness and may have made peace with anticipated death, while family members may be focused on loss and may urge additional interventions. In such a scenario, it can be helpful to steer conversations back to what the patient wants and what is in her best interest. It is also important to remember that family dynamics are complex and what may be most important to the patient at that time, despite feeling prepared for death, is to honor the family request.

Goal setting via surrogates adds an additional layer of complexity. The physician's task in this setting is to help surrogates focus on the patient's goals, whether previously stated or inferred, rather than the surrogate's goals. This can be accomplished by hypothetically "bringing the patient into the conversation" using the following language:

To the Patient: What do you hope for the most, if your time is limited? When you think about the future, what worries you the most?

To the Surrogate: If your loved one was sitting here with us, listening to what we just discussed, what would he say?

Physicians must be able to identify what is medically reasonable and help provide information so that patients and families can understand and accept what may or may not be medically possible or beneficial. The impact of certain interventions may be difficult to foresee, and in such a case it can be helpful to agree on a predetermined time frame in which to measure the outcomes of a proposed plan of action in relation to patient goals.

Goals of care and the decision-making process are as dynamic as the trajectory of illness, so reassessment and continued communication are crucial to maintaining patient-centered care.

Clinical Situation

Juanita's Case Continues (continued from page 45)

It is 1 week later and you are seeing Juanita in your palliative care office. You spoke with the oncologist this morning, who tells you that further testing has revealed locally advanced, nonresectable disease. As Juanita has excellent performance status, the oncologist recommends first-line chemotherapy with gemcitabine. The oncologist met with Juanita and her husband yesterday to discuss the diagnosis, expected disease trajectory, and treatment options. Juanita and her husband requested time to think about their options and scheduled follow-up with the oncologist next week.

As you prepare for your meeting with Juanita and her husband, you think about ways to help them consider the treatment options. You know there is no right decision in this setting, and the decision should be made within the context of what is important to Juanita and her family. You plan to ask the following questions to help explore Juanita's goals and preferences for her medical care (**Table 13**).

Case continues on page 55

Table 13. Identifying Goals, Values, and Preferences

Skill	Language
Understanding the patient's cognitive and emotional perspective of her illness.	Tell me more about your understanding of your illness.
	Tell me more about how you are feeling about your illness.
	Tell me more about how you are making sense of all of this.
Understanding the impact of the illness on the patient's life.	Tell me more about how your illness is impacting your life.
	What is the hardest part of what is going on right now for you and your family?
Eliciting the patient's hope and worry for the future.	When you think about the future, what concerns you the most?
	What do you hope for the most if your time is limited? or What is most important to you if your time is limited?

Reframing Goals

There are times during the course of serious illness when patient-identified goals of medical care need to be redefined in the face of a changing clinical landscape, such as cancer progressing despite anticancer treatments. There are other times when patient-identified goals of medical care are not possible within the clinical context (eg, hoping for a cure despite metastatic disease). In these scenarios, it is the physician's job to help patients reframe their goals of medical care to those that are achievable and beneficial while carefully balancing hope with realism. This conversation requires disrupting patients from their comfort zone (eg, life with cancer on chemotherapy) and helping patients reconfigure to a new norm (eg, life with cancer without chemotherapy and limited life expectancy).[171] **Table 14** provides a talking map that can facilitate such conversations.[179]

Table 14. REMAP[178]

Task	Description	Language
Reframe the status quo	Examine why things are currently not proceeding as everyone hoped.	"Given this news, it seems like a good time to talk about what to do now." "We're in a different place."
Expect **E**motion and **E**mpathize	Transitions are difficult; expect patients to have an emotional reaction to the changes. Help to process this change through empathic displays.	"It's hard to deal with all this." "I can see you are really concerned about…" "Tell me more about that; what are you worried about?" "Is it okay for us to talk about what this means?"
Map the future	Explore patient goals and values to help plan for the "new" future.	"Given this situation, what's most important for you?" "When you think about the future, are there things you want to do?" "As you think toward the future, what concerns you?"
Align with the patient's values	Reframe the future in the context of what the patient finds most important.	"As I listen to you, it sounds like the most important things are…"
Plan medical treatments that match values	Provide a clear recommendation on how patient goals may be achieved.	"Here's what I can do now that will help you do those important things."

Adapted from Addressing Goals of Care: "REMAP," by VitalTalk, http://www.vitaltalk.org/sites/default/files/quick-guides/REMAPforVitaltalkV1.0.pdf, Accessed April 24, 2017. ©2017 VitalTalk. Adapted with permission.

💡 Statements to Reframe Unrealistic Goals for Medical Care

A patient with metastatic cancer and a prognosis of months states her goal is to watch her daughter graduate from high school next year.

"I am hoping, as you are, that the treatment works to slow your disease so that you are able to celebrate your daughter's achievement. I am worried that you may become much sicker before this happens. Are you willing to talk about what it may look like if it doesn't work as we would like? In any case, I will continue to work with you to ensure that you are well taken care of."

When patient-identified goals of medical care are unrealistic within the clinical context, this is usually the result of poor prognostic awareness. Communication strategies that encourage patients to hope while also preparing for an undesired outcome can be helpful.[180]

Achieving a Shared Decision

Shared decision making allows the patient's values and preferences and the physician's clinical knowledge and expertise to lead the two parties to a joint decision for care. In this model, as Kon explains, there exists a continuum of shared decision-making, ranging from patient driven to physician driven with different levels of partnership throughout.[47] Unlike discussions regarding nonurgent procedures, medical decision making can be overwhelming for seriously ill patients at the end of life when the "right" is ambiguous and decisions are heavily laden with emotion. Often, when decisions are emotionally complex and concern imminent death, patients and families find it useful for the physician to make a clear recommendation. Quill and Brody describe this technique as "enhanced autonomy."[181] In this scenario, the physician's expert opinion enhances the patient's autonomous choice by relieving the burden of an emotionally laden decision while still allowing the patient or family to reject the recommendation. Quill and Brody recommend this approach as an alternative to what they call "independent choice," where the patient and family are left to make a clinical decision based only on statistical odds without the benefit of a professional opinion. Although the model of independent choice maximizes patient and family control, it does so at the expense of clinical competence. For the model of enhanced autonomy to be most successful, a recommendation framed within the context of patient-specific goals and values should be made only after asking permission, and after sharing with the patient and family that there may not be any "right" decision. It is important to check in with patients to assess their response to the recommendation (see **Table 15**).

Shared decision making is a collaborative effort between physician and patient to develop a medically appropriate care plan that is consistent with a patient's values and goals. Shared decision making relies upon a knowledgeable physician (one who is well versed in the medical facts and treatment options), an informed patient (one with solid prognostic awareness), and a

Table 15. Sample Statements for Shared Decision Making

Ask permission	Would it be okay if I made a recommendation based on what we discussed today?
Make a patient-centered recommendation	You have told me that the most important consideration for you right now is spending time with the people you love. Recently the chemotherapy has been making you too sick to engage with and enjoy your loved ones. The goal of the palliative chemotherapy is to improve your quality of life. It appears it is no longer achieving this goal; therefore, I think stopping chemotherapy would be appropriate at this time.
Assess patient response	What reactions do you have to my recommendation?

mutual understanding of the patient's values, preferences, and realistic goals of medical care. A deficiency in any of these components will result in a communication breakdown and fail to achieve a shared decision.

For some patients, the dialogue needed to identify prognostic awareness and goals for the future is not possible. This may be due to cognitive impairment, medical naïveté, severe anxiety, magical thinking, or a culture that defers to authority, among other factors.[182] These patients may exhibit maladaptive coping mechanisms that can be identified by a protracted emotional response to open-ended questions. These responses can include such statements as "You should know, you're the doctor!" or "I don't know, they don't tell me anything!" A patient may fixate on one point, such as "I don't understand why you can't just operate to remove the cancer." In this setting, open-ended questions and unlimited care options may cause more suffering by increasing the burden of the decision and possibly leading to nonbeneficial care. An approach coined "palliative paternalism" has been described, where the physician, after recognizing maladaptive coping, limits open-ended questions and utilizes well-informed, discrete, concrete options. In this situation, the physician determines the appropriate level of patient autonomy and follows with a declarative statement about the medical situation. The physician continues to pause and observe the reaction, providing empathetic statements. Each time an adaptive response is given, the physician can follow with an open-ended question; however, when a maladaptive response is given, the physician follows with a declarative statement. In this way, the physician can determine where on the shared decision-making continuum (**Figure 2**) the patient feels most comfortable.

Figure 2. Shared Decision-Making Continuum[47]

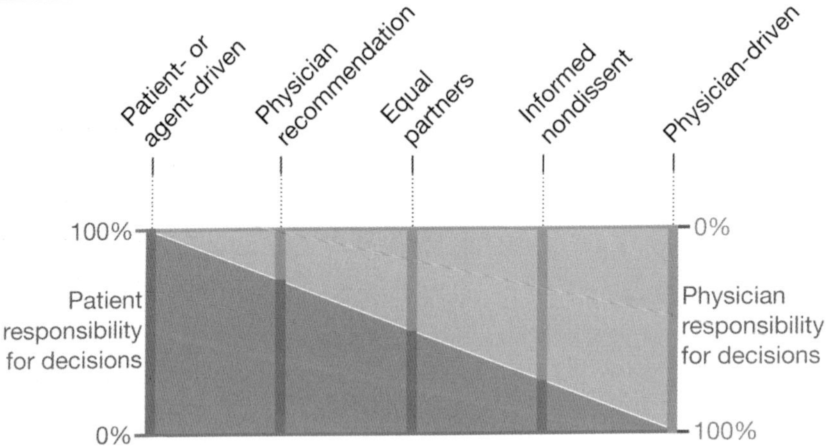

From "The shared decision-making continuum," by A Kon, JAMA. 2010 Aug 25;304(8):903-4. © 2010 American Medical Association. Reproduced with permission. All rights reserved.

Clinical Situation

Juanita's Case Continues (continued from page 51)

Juanita presents for a follow-up visit. Through the questions you prepared to elicit her goals and preferences for medical care, you learn that Juanita is saddened and shocked by the recent news that she has incurable cancer that will significantly shorten her life. She is coping through the loving support of her family and knowledge that "God will provide." With regard to the future, she worries most about her family—both their sadness and not being able to perform in her role as the "strong mother" who "takes care of everyone." In addition, she worries about pain and about being a burden to her family as her disease progresses. She hopes to remain independent and pain free, allowing her to provide for her family for as long as possible.

The oncologist has told you that the intent of palliative chemotherapy is to control the spread of disease, which will hopefully provide symptom control and preserve function. The oncologist feels a trial of palliative chemotherapy would be a reasonable option for Juanita based on her disease and functional status.

Juanita and her husband tell you they have been struggling to decide about how to proceed with treatment. They ask for your advice. Based on Juanita's goals and your knowledge of the medical facts, you make the following recommendation:

The Conversation	Specific Strategies and Skills
You: Juanita, I can see that you have been struggling to decide how to proceed with treatment.	Respond to the patient's feelings (**N**URSE [Name]).
Juanita: Yes, you are right. I've been back and forth a hundred times.	
You: This is understandable. It is normal for these decisions to be overwhelming and even confusing.	Respond to the patient's feelings (Normalizing).
Juanita: It's good to know I'm not the only one who feels this way.	
You: You are definitely experiencing very normal feelings. We have discussed a lot, both about your cancer and about what is most important to you. Would it be helpful if I made a recommendation based on what we have discussed here today?	Shared decision making: ask permission to provide a recommendation.
Juanita *(looking relieved)*: Oh, yes. That would be very helpful. I just want to be sure I am making the right decision.	

You: I'm not sure there is a right or wrong decision in this situation, only what feels most comfortable for you and your family. I am here to help you figure out what that may be.

Juanita: Thank you. It is comforting to know you will be here to help us. So, what do you think would be best for me?

You: You have told me that being able to continue taking care of your family is most important to you right now. The goal of the palliative chemotherapy is to improve your quality of life by controlling symptoms and preserving function. These are all things necessary for you to continue providing for your family. *(Pause.)*

Therefore, I think a trial of chemotherapy would be appropriate to help you achieve your goals. *(Pause.)*

It is possible that the treatments may not work in the way we hope. It is possible that the treatments could make you sicker. We can and should stop the chemotherapy at any time if the treatments are not helping you to reach your goals. *(Allow a period of silence to let Juanita absorb the recommendation.)*

You: What reactions do you have to my recommendation?

Juanita: That makes a lot of sense to me. I think trying the chemotherapy makes sense.

You: Can you summarize for me what we discussed here today?

Juanita: I need to be around to take care of my family for as long as possible. The treatments are supposed to help me do that. If it doesn't, if the chemotherapy actually makes me feel worse, we can stop it at any time.

You: That's right, Juanita. I will be here with you throughout your treatments, and we can continue to evaluate the benefit of your treatments together. I will call you next week after your first treatment.

Respond to the patient's feelings (NUR**S**E [Support]).

Shared decision making: make a patient-centered recommendation (small steps and stop frequently).

Respond to the patient's feelings (therapeutic silence).

Shared decision making: assess patient response.

Make a plan: summarize the interview.

Respond to the patient's feelings (NUR**S**E [Support]).

Make a plan (make a contract).

Case continues on page 65

Communicating Prognosis

Whenever serious sickness or injury strikes and your body or mind breaks down, the vital questions are the same: What is your understanding of the situation and its potential outcomes? What are your fears and what are your hopes? What are the trade-offs you are willing to make and not willing to make? And what is the course of action that best serves this understanding?

—Atul Gawande, MD[183]

Gauging Prognostic Awareness

Physicians often give inadequate information about prognosis.[184,185] Either it is not discussed,[186] or physicians will give overly optimistic predictions.[187] In one study, even when asked, physicians would provide a truthful prognostic estimate in only about one-third of cases.[188] Prognostic discussions are particularly rare when disease is nonmalignant,[189] during phase 1 trials,[190] and in palliative chemotherapy settings.[191] When prognosis is discussed, it is often introduced in the context of whether a treatment will work[192] or addressed late in the course when all treatment options have been exhausted.[193] Physicians primarily describe prognosis in qualitative terms, rarely ask if family members want to hear the news, and often fail to check understanding.[194] Physicians may not want to discuss prognosis for fear that truthful communication about limited prognosis may destroy hope. Physician reluctance to discuss prognosis is further complicated by patient optimism bias and the perception that physicians who present positive prognostic information are more compassionate.[195] Patients, however, do not find withholding prognosis an acceptable means to maintain hope.[161] Rather, they draw hope from a doctor who appears up to date, knowledgeable, and confident and who promises that symptoms will be controlled.[196]

Patients generally want to know their prognosis[160] and have legitimate needs for the information. Knowing their prognosis allows patients to prioritize their plans for the future[161] and make medical decisions. Patients who have an accurate understanding of prognosis are less likely to want aggressive end-of-life care.[197,198] Patients who have a poor understanding of prognosis are less likely to engage in end-of-life planning, such as discussing care preferences with family members.[199]

Most family members also want to know the prognosis for similar planning reasons. Interestingly, families may doubt the physician's ability to prognosticate[200] and tend to use the physician's estimate of prognosis as only one factor as they predict how long their loved one will live, giving equal or greater weight to factors such as the patient's perceived willingness to fight and how they responded to prior illnesses.[201] Nevertheless, families find the physician's opinion valuable and want to hear it.[200]

Although most patients and families want to talk about prognosis, they generally want to negotiate how and when it is discussed.[202] Unfortunately, there is no way to know when a patient wants to have this discussion. Disease severity does not predict interest in discussing end-of-life issues.[203] The only way for a clinician to know is to ask. One phrase proposed in the literature is "How much do you want to know about the future?"[204] In response to this question, patients will either want to know, not want to know, or be ambivalent. For those who do not want to know, the clinician should explore their reasoning. Often such a response is based on the difficult emotions associated with the topic, and addressing these emotions can help move the conversation forward. If, however, there is a desire not to know for cultural or other reasons, the physician must decide if knowing this information will influence decision making. If it will, patients may allow the physician to convey the information to a family member or other surrogate decision maker. If the patient is ambivalent, naming this ambivalence and exploring the underlying cognitive and emotional issues may be helpful.

If the patient agrees to hear the prognosis or initiates the question, the physician should proceed with a thoughtful discussion of the topic.[166] If the patient brings up the question, the physician should ask for clarification about goals and expectations and not immediately provide specific time frames. The patient may be seeking information regarding a specific future event rather than a time frame of weeks or months. It can also be helpful to ask what the patient has heard or knows about the prognosis because this information may frame the rest of the discussion. The ask-tell-ask approach (Table 4) is helpful here.[166] The following dialogue serves as an example of assessing prognostic awareness:

Physician: What have you been told about your prognosis?

Patient: Not much at all.

Physician: What is your sense of how much time you have?

Patient: I don't know.

Physician: Would it be helpful for you if I shared my thoughts on your prognosis?

Patient: Yes, I want to know. How long have I got?

OR

Patient: No, I don't think I want to hear that right now.

Physician: That's absolutely fine. Is there someone you'd like me to talk to instead?

Discussing Prognosis

When giving prognostic information, physicians should provide clear and straightforward estimates and ensure that patients understand what they have been told. Patients tend to overestimate their prognosis,[205] and unless the physician is direct in providing a realistic estimate, concordance between the patient and the physician's perception remains poor.[66] Surrogate optimism bias can be tempered by framing decisions as the patient's choice instead of the surrogate's decision and by describing interventions like cardiopulmonary resuscitation (CPR) in less technical terms.[206] Physicians should also ensure consistency in prognostic information from different team members and involve the family if appropriate.[207] Although it is unclear whether it is better to give qualitative or quantitative estimates[208] at the end of life, many practitioners find it best to give ranges of time such as hours to days, days to weeks, weeks to months, or several months to a year or so. The physician can remain aligned with the patient psychologically by acknowledging that all estimates are uncertain. Acknowledging uncertainty and the communication behaviors that go along with it have been associated with increased patient satisfaction.[209] Patients and surrogates recognize there is uncertainty at the end of life but still find the prognostic estimates helpful[210] and use communication as their main means to manage this uncertainty.[211] It is often helpful to acknowledge that a particular patient may live longer or shorter than average estimates. While acknowledging that no one can accurately predict the future, physicians can encourage patients to revise unrealistic goals, go on trips when they are feeling well enough to do so, visit with family, and say all they want to say and do all the things they want to accomplish before dying.[212] Such responses convey important information, maintain hope, and encourage patients to complete the developmental tasks of dying[213] (see *UNIPAC 2*). The following dialogue serves as an example of a disclosure of prognosis:

Patient: How long have I got?

Physician: It sounds like you are asking about how much time you have left to live. Is that correct? (Patient nods.) What have you been told about your prognosis?

Patient: Not much at all.

Physician: What is your sense of how much time you have?

Patient: I don't know.

Physician: No one can predict life expectancy exactly. There is always a lot of uncertainty, and we can't say for sure how your disease will progress. Based on the medical indications and your situation, you are likely to live for a few more weeks and maybe as long as a couple of months.

Patient: So it's really that bad?

Physician: I sense this is not what you were expecting to hear.

Patient: I… I thought I would have more time.

Physician: I wish things were different too, and I want you to know I'll be here to support you and your family. What are some of the things that are important to you in the time you have?

Discussing Prognosis

Important points to remember when giving life expectancy estimates include the following:

- Avoid unwarranted optimism or overestimation. Give patients and families a general time frame that is as accurate as possible.
- Use the patient's activity level and ability to perform activities of daily living as the best prognostic indicator.[214] Several prognostic tools also are available to help guide determination of prognosis (see *UNIPAC 1*).[215]
- Respond to emotion with empathy. Use silence strategically.
- Encourage patients and families to use their remaining time to complete important tasks (see *UNIPAC 2*).

Denial and the Patient

Patients usually react to distressing events with characteristic responses formed over the course of a lifetime. Examples of responses include anger, denial, a desire for more information, optimism, acceptance, and certainty that the worst will occur.[216] When patients are faced with news of a life-threatening illness, denial is one of the most common reactions. However, the level of denial is rarely consistent; it usually waxes and wanes throughout the course of an illness based on the patient's ability to accept the implications of the diagnosis. Most of the time patients experience several conflicting emotions simultaneously (eg, denial and anger, fear and hope, or a mix of optimism and despair), all of which are likely to resurface throughout the course of the illness.[216]

A patient's psychological defenses should be respected whenever possible because they are based on lifelong patterns of coping with the exigencies of life. Efforts to break down a patient's deep-seated denial more than likely reflect the needs of the caregiver, not the patient, and should be attempted by psychiatrists only when absolutely necessary. At the same time, it is clear that a high degree of denial presents challenges for the team because it complicates planning for the future, often results in underreporting of pain and other distressing symptoms, and irritates family members and caregivers, which affects their interactions with the patient.[217,218]

Frequently what appears to be denial may simply represent a different narrative the patient has constructed to understand his or her illness. Exploring this narrative to better understand the patient perspective may be the most fruitful approach and may even help with physical symptom control.[219,220]

Behaviors That Appear Unreasonable

Instead of immediately labeling patients "unreasonable" or "in denial" when their expectations do not align with the medical team's expectations, first ask yourself the following questions:

- Why is this person asking for something that I feel is unreasonable?
- Why do I feel that this person is in denial?
- How can I better understand this person's perspective? Am I missing part of the story?
- Am I communicating with this person in the best way possible, based on his communication style and not my own?

Clinical Situation

Ethel

Ethel is an 80-year-old woman with advanced ischemic heart failure. She has dyspnea at rest and is not a candidate for any intervention including transplant or a ventricular assist device. She has bilateral leg pain from peripheral vascular disease, and you are asked to help manage her pain. You are specifically told to not discuss goals of care. When you approach the room, the patient's son jumps up and meets you before you can come through the door. He tells you that the family has decided to not tell the patient how sick she is, so he asks that you not mention any bad news. You tell him you have been asked to help with the pain, so he cautiously allows you to enter the room. After talking with the patient for a while, she mentions how sick she feels and how tired she is of going back and forth between home and the hospital. Her son reassures her that this time they will get her better so she can get back to her old self. The patient does not seem to believe him but reluctantly becomes quiet. You finish your exam and make some proposals regarding pain control and then leave, promising to return tomorrow. The son steps into the hallway with you and says that they know she is dying but don't see the value in taking away her hope.

- How do you respond to a family request for nondisclosure of information?

- What is the best way to balance your desires to advocate for the patient and be a good consultant who does not overstep bounds?

- Do patients generally want to know their prognosis? Does knowledge of prognosis "take away hope?"

Denial and the Family

Best practice dictates that coherent patients always should be asked about their preferences for receiving medical information. Patients may indicate that they wish to receive all information alone, to receive information with another person, or for information to be shared with a relative or friend rather than shared directly. Ten to twenty percent of adult patients do not wish to know their prognosis.[204] Clinicians should also inquire whether anyone besides the patient can receive medical information. Sometimes, however, patients are not coherent, and news of a terminal condition is first disclosed to family members. In other situations, such as the one in Ethel Miller's case above, family members sense a serious illness and intervene before any discussion can occur. In these situations, family members may want to withhold the information from the patient.[68] When physicians comply with such requests, they risk reinforcing the mistaken notion that death and dying are too frightening and horrible to discuss, and they exclude patients from participating in healthcare decisions and completing the developmental tasks of the dying[213] (see *UNIPAC 2*). Physicians should respond to such requests for nondisclosure of information with compassion and explore the underlying concerns. Although there may be a cultural reason to not disclose the information, the request usually reflects the family's fears and concerns about death and their desire to protect the patient.[221] The physician can use this as an opportunity to educate family members about the adverse effects of withholding information, model effective communication about death-related issues, and learn about cultural differences about communication. **Table 16** lists strategies that encourage communication about dying between patients and their families[222] and help clinicians respond to requests for nondisclosure of information.

Sometimes, despite open communication and nonjudgmental exploration with the family, a physician is put in a difficult situation in which the family refuses disclosure to the patient. The physician, however, has an ethical obligation to refrain from lying to patients or withholding information requested by patients. In this setting, it is often helpful to use a strategy called *informed refusal*, by which the physician asks the patient how she would like to handle information about her illness.[74] Many patients will decide to hear the information even if it is not the cultural norm the family assumes. In fact, caregivers have been shown to be poor at predicting what the patient would want to know,[223] and informed patients have better expectations for the future than those who are not informed.[155]

The "Some-Other" Technique

"Some people like to know all the details of their test results and their diagnosis; others prefer that this information be shared with their family instead. There is no right or wrong approach. What is your preference for receiving information?"

OR

"Some people want to be directly involved in the decision-making process; others would rather have their family make healthcare decisions for them. There is no right or wrong. What is your preference for decision-making?"

Troubleshooting Prognosis

The use of empathetic communication skills is essential when providing prognostic information, and many of these skills are discussed in the chapter Communicating Serious News (pages 29-47). Two additional communication tools that help promote prognostic awareness while attending to the patient's emotional and coping needs are "hope and worry" and "I wish" statements.[8]

The "hope and worry" skill is a way to align with a patient's goals while expressing concern and empathetically exploring what might happen if these goals are not achieved. Often patients and families hope for outcomes that are seen as unreasonable to the medical team.

Table 16. Strategies for Responding to Requests for Nondisclosure of Information

Normalize Concerns Acknowledge the difficulty of talking about a serious illness.	"On a very primitive level, most people believe that death can be prevented by not talking about it—saying the words makes it a reality."
Assess Gentle but direct questions can elicit additional clues about the family's coping styles and their underlying fears.	"What are some of your concerns about sharing this information with your mother?" "What is likely to happen if the information is not shared?" "What is likely to happen if the information is shared?"
Educate/Explore Provide information about the benefits of communicating with patients.	"Most patients with terminal illness know they are dying." "Most dying patients want more information about their diagnosis and prognosis than anyone realizes." "Most dying patients want to talk about death-related concerns." "Withholding information could affect your mother's trust in her physicians and family members." "Withholding information could isolate your mother and prevent her from planning for the future and making treatment-related decisions." "Ethically, physicians cannot refuse to share information with patients if they want to know." "There is no substitute for saying goodbye; it is important for the patient and critical for the surviving family."[142]
Respond with Empathy Acknowledge family concerns.	"I can't imagine how hard it must be to talk about death and dying." "I wonder if you are feeling anxious about your mother knowing her prognosis." "It's clear how much you love your mother. You are an amazing advocate for her."
Negotiate Information Sharing Set expectations and discuss how information will be shared.	"Perhaps we can see how much information your mother wants to know?" "If she wants to know, I will be as sensitive as possible to your concerns about disclosing her prognosis and will share the information respectfully." "If she does not want to know, then we will not share this information with her and instead will speak directly with you."

Instead of labeling these hopes as unreasonable, a gentle exploration of the root of this hope may be more effective. To gauge prognostic awareness and troubleshoot someone's disbelief in a given prognosis, a healthcare provider may ask, "We have talked about how much time may be left, and I'm sensing you feel something different. What are the things you are hoping for, and what are some of the things you are worried about?" Another way of framing this is to "hope for the best, and prepare for the worst."[172]

Similarly an "I wish" statement is a way of aligning the goals of the healthcare team with the goals of the patient while implying that such a goal is unlikely to occur.[170] It is an empathetic communication strategy that aligns goals and expectations without judgment and may serve as a way to build trust while fostering the shared humanity between clinician and patient. One key in using an "I wish" statement is to follow it with a strategic use of silence. Resist the urge to speak, or say "I wish… but." Instead stay silent and see what the patient says. An example of an "I wish" statement is "I wish I could tell you precisely how much time you have left."

Table 17 provides several other examples of "hope and worry" and "I wish" statements.

Table 17. "Hope and Worry" and "I Wish" Statements

Hope and Worry

"It sounds like you are hoping your father will walk again, and the doctors are worried this won't happen. Have you thought about what your father would say if he is not able to walk again?"

"It sounds like you are hoping this chemotherapy will cure your cancer, and I am hoping for the same. Is there anything you are worried about?"

I Wish

"I wish there was a way to cure your cancer."

"It sounds like you are hoping for a new chemotherapy treatment. I really wish there was another medication we could use to treat your cancer."

Communicating with Loved Ones

Although the individual is the unit of treatment, the family is the unit of understanding. According to family systems theory, each system or subsystem is always part of a larger system, whether it begins with the cardiovascular system, the whole body system, the whole person system, or the whole family system. Each of these systems, or subsystems, is in constant interaction with all other smaller subsystems that are within it, as well as in constant interaction with the larger supra-system of the environment that is around it.[122]

—Williamson and Noel

The family conference is a key component of communication during end-of-life care.[224] It is used perhaps most prominently in the intensive care unit (ICU) but is also common on general hospital units, in the clinic, and in patient homes. Leading a family conference can be difficult and requires a unique set of skills that often are not taught.[16] If conducted well, it can be a powerful tool.

One study showed that implementing a system of regularly scheduled, well-conducted family meetings in the ICU resulted in a decreased length of stay without an increase in mortality.[18,225] Another study randomized surrogates to receive either routine interactions or a bereavement brochure and a proactive end-of-life family conference during which many of the communication techniques described in this book would be used. The family members in the conference group were found to have fewer symptoms of anxiety, depression, and posttraumatic stress disorder.[226]

Often, however, family conferences are conducted poorly,[227] which can lead to impaired decision making and long-term consequences for the family, including a significant risk of posttraumatic stress disorder.[228] To participate effectively, physicians should understand the basics of family systems theory, develop a sense of the family's beliefs and behaviors, and recognize the family's current stage of development. Toward that end, this section will begin with an explanation of family systems theory and end with specific recommendations for how to conduct a family meeting and a review of challenges often faced in these situations.

Clinical Situation

Juanita's Case Continues (continued from page 56)

Juanita's oncologist comes to you to ask for your help. Juanita has now been on palliative chemotherapy for 8 weeks, and recent imaging shows that her cancer has progressed. She is tolerating the therapy with preserved functional status and good symptom control. Juanita and her family are trying to decide whether to pursue an alternate palliative chemotherapy option or a care plan more focused on comfort. Her husband is an engineer and takes vigorous notes during all meetings. She also has three children: a nurse and two engineers. They are trying to decide whether to initiate chemotherapy. Juanita is hesitant and one of her daughters is supportive, but her husband, son, and other daughter believe she should do everything possible. The oncology team had met with them last week to discuss treatment and, according to the social worker, "it was a disaster." The differences in opinions escalated into heated arguments, and the oncologist decided to end the meeting and meet again today so everyone could calm down. Because you are "good with families who experience conflict," she asks if you would mind helping to facilitate the meeting. You agree and ask to spend some time discussing the case with the oncologist and the social worker before going in to see the patient. During this discussion, the social worker mentions that the family is very enmeshed and has a closed family system.

> What is the difference between an enmeshed and a disengaged family system?

> What is the difference between a closed and open family system, and how might this difference influence the upcoming discussion?

> You believe a recommendation from the physician might help resolve the disagreement, but how can you make a recommendation that does not impose your personal values? Will such a recommendation be welcome?

> What would be the best way to respond to the husband and children's request to "do everything?"

Case continues on page 77

Family Systems Theory

Instead of viewing a person as an individual unit, family systems theory views the individual as "one part of a larger (emotional) system of the family, with the family seen as the whole."[122] Family systems theory suggests that a patient's actions are best understood within the context of the family system, which sets rules about communication and interaction. Remember that individuals may have different definitions of what a family entails. It is always important to ask what constitutes an individual's family rather than assume a traditional construct. In general, family systems theory includes the following basic concepts:[122]

- The whole is greater than the sum of the parts. For example, a person is more than the sum of various bodily systems.
- Whatever affects the system as a whole affects each part. For example, morphine affects not only the sensory system but also the gastrointestinal and cognitive systems and the patient's ability to interact with family and friends.

- A change in any part of a system affects every part of the system and the system as a whole. For example, pain relief positively benefits not only the patient but also the entire family system.

Regardless of a system's size or complexity (whether it is one person or an entire family), systems are dynamic. They develop rules, roles, and patterns of behavior to sustain them. Because systems tend to view any change as a threat to their continued existence, they may fear even beneficial changes and rely on entrenched behavior patterns, even when those behaviors are no longer helpful.

Family systems must constantly adjust to internal stressors (eg, the birth of a child or a serious illness) and external stressors (eg, job loss, cultural or religious discrimination, lack of access to health care). When profound stressors such as a terminal illness and the death of a family member occur, the entire family system may be thrown out of balance. The stresses associated with adaptation may trigger or exacerbate long-standing family issues related to beliefs, roles, rules, and unresolved earlier losses, and can impact coping and bereavement.[216]

The Family Life Cycle

Like any other system, traditional families experience the following developmental stages:
- new couple
- family with young child(ren)
- family with adolescent(s)
- family with children leaving home
- aging family dealing with retirement, serious illness
- death of one parent or partner, and then the other.

Whether changes are expected and welcomed (eg, birth of child) or unexpected and feared (eg, job loss, divorce, serious illness), they require major adjustments in the family members' roles and functions. When the death of a family member occurs amid a new developmental stage, the combined stress of adjusting to the death and the developmental stage is likely to pose tremendous challenges for the entire family system.

Family Interaction Models

Enmeshed or Disengaged

Minuchin characterized family systems as enmeshed or disengaged.[229] When families are enmeshed, their tightly woven relationships present an almost impenetrable barrier to the outside world. The identities of enmeshed family members are so interconnected with each other and with the family system as a whole that the death of one member creates particularly difficult identity and self-esteem problems for survivors. Enmeshed families may find it difficult to communicate with or accept help from outsiders because of unspoken rules prohibiting sharing information with strangers.

Disengaged families represent the other extreme. They are so separate from one another that there is little mutual dependence, little sharing of functions and roles, and limited emotional support. Family bonds may appear nonexistent, and team members may have difficulty distinguishing family members from visitors and friends. However, when serious illness occurs, disengaged families may temporarily regroup and erect barriers between the family and the outside world.

The terms *enmeshed* and *disengaged* do not always imply dysfunction. All families exist somewhere on a continuum of enmeshed and disengaged interaction according to their needs. Functional enmeshment is appropriate in certain situations. For example, when an infant is born, the tightly woven interdependent connections between the parents and child help ensure the child's survival. When a family member is dying, family members often assume the patient's responsibilities and provide much more physical and emotional support than usual, thereby protecting the patient until death occurs.

Closed or Open

Satir described family systems as open or closed, depending on the family's communication patterns, rules, and relationships with the outside world.[230] An *open* family system's permeable boundaries and encouragement of supportive relationships with the outside world generally allow greater access to patients and family members. *Closed* family systems, like other closed groups, whether social, religious, or work related, establish rigid boundaries between their members and outsiders, presenting challenges for hospice and palliative care teams. **Table 18** describes the characteristics of open and closed family systems.[230]

Although open family systems are better able to adapt to changing situations than closed family systems, open families also experience tremendous stress as members adapt to the terminal illness and death of a family member. For physicians, the important point to remember is that a family's beliefs and patterns of behavior influence its willingness to ask for and accept help, its ability to communicate about illness and death, its willingness to care for the dying person, and its response to the death of one of its members.

Family Subsystems

Within families, smaller subsystems exist based on age (adults or children), sex (mothers and daughters), areas of interest (reading or fishing), or function (subgroups of grandparents, parents, or siblings). Other family subsystems include the following[97,230]:

- Pairs—Each pair has a role name, such as spouse-spouse, partner-partner, parent-child, sibling-sibling, and so forth. Families with rigid beliefs are likely to experience particular difficulty when confronted with change; for example, a strict belief that only wives cook leads to adjustment difficulties when the wife becomes too ill to cook.
- Triangles—Families with more than two members contain subsystems of triangles. A family of five members includes 30 triangles, including father-mother-first son,

Table 18. Characteristics of Open and Closed Family Systems

Open	Closed
Characteristics	
Views change as normal, inevitable, and desirable.	Change is feared and resisted.
Encourages supportive relationships with the outside world.	Restricts contact or transactions with the outside world.
Uses direct, clear, and specific communication.	Uses indirect, unclear, and nonspecific communication.
Uses flexible rules to govern the family's behavior.	Uses covert rules that don't change according to family needs.
Encourages communication and comments about family rules and beliefs.	Prohibits comments about family rules and beliefs.
Self-worth is primary; power and performance are secondary.	Self-worth is secondary to power and performance.
Actions represent one's beliefs.	Actions are subject to the whims of the "boss."
Rules and Beliefs	
Mistakes are normal and okay.	Never make mistakes.
Feelings are important.	Don't raise your voice.
We can work it out.	Don't talk about _____ 's illness or death.
You are a special person.	Children must be protected from painful experiences (eg, funerals).
It is okay to ask for what you want.	Asking for what you want is selfish.
We can talk about our problems with each other and with the outside world.	We can't talk about or acknowledge our family secrets.
	Relationships must be regulated by force or punishment.
	There is one right way, and the person with the most power is the only one who knows it.
	Those in authority know what is best for you.

father-mother-daughter, and father-first son-daughter. Because of the number of triangles existing in each family, dysfunctional relationships challenge the entire family system; for example, when parents experience relationship difficulties, one of them may turn to a young child or to an outside affair for emotional support instead of seeking professional help or talking with friends.
- Coalitions—*Coalitions* are subsystems that form to serve a special purpose. During a terminal illness, they commonly form around issues such as the location of care; for example, one coalition may insist the patient remain at home, but another insists the patient move to a nursing facility.

Family Responses to Terminal Illness and Death

A family system's response to the profound illness and death of one of its members is affected by the system's beliefs and behavior patterns, including family roles, rules, and level of intimacy.

Family Roles

When one member of a family system becomes profoundly ill or dies, other family members must assume new roles and responsibilities. The amount of disruption experienced by the family system is likely to be affected by the following[97]:

- Family position held by the individual. If the individual is the family's only child, the parents will experience tremendous stress as they adjust to the state of childlessness.
- Number and type of roles held by the individual. If the individual is the family's only wage earner or main communicator, remaining family members are likely to experience significant stress as they learn to cope with financial issues or communicate directly with one another instead of through the communicator.
- Ability of family members to perform tasks essential to family life. If illness, disability, or lack of education and skills interferes with the family's ability to fill a vacant role, the system will experience significant stress until family members adjust or find outside help.
- Degree of scapegoating. Dysfunctional families often identify one family member as the problem person and blame that person for all of the family's problems. By focusing on problems caused by the scapegoat instead of its own systemic problems, the family tries to avoid change, a much-feared process that can result in the "death" of dysfunctional but familiar behavior patterns.

Family Rules

When one member of a family system becomes profoundly ill, adjustments in family rules are usually required. For example, a family rule against accepting outside help must be relaxed if the family is to receive financial help from the Medicare hospice benefit. The drug-abuse prevention slogan "just say no" may result in family rules that prohibit drug use; these families must adapt if the patient requires medication to relieve pain. A rule prohibiting outsiders in the home must also be relaxed to allow home care.

Intimacy Patterns
When death occurs, family members may become so isolated in their own grief that they may be unable to emotionally support themselves or other members of the family. The family system then requires temporary support from a bereavement team until adequate functioning is restored. The stresses associated with a terminal illness and death may strengthen emotional ties among family members, but the stresses also can cause disintegration of family relationships. Families may temporarily change their pattern of relating during the illness but are likely to revert to their former patterns after the death occurs.

When it comes to the issue of touch, patient needs vary. Some seriously ill patients suffer from a lack of touch and want the emotional reassurance and healing that caring touch provides. Others do not want to be touched at all. In some specific populations, such as patients with end-stage dementia, touch can be therapeutic.[231]

Protracted illness and inpatient care often interfere with a couple's privacy needs. Some couples want privacy for long talks, cuddling, prayer, or sexual intimacy. Physicians should encourage them to establish private times, particularly during inpatient stays. Other couples are distressed by intimacy and fear the personal aspects of home care. Such patients may not want family members, including spouses, to touch them or provide personal care. In any case, the patient's wishes should be respected.

Facilitating Family Conferences
Careful planning is essential for effective family conferences. Before the conference, the physician should confer with other members of the interdisciplinary team and decide the following:
- Which family members and professional staff will participate in the conference?
- Do individual issues exist that must be addressed one on one before the conference?
- Where and when will the conference take place? Which room can comfortably accommodate participants? What time is most convenient for family members?
- Which professional staff members will assume responsibility for various aspects of the conference? Who will invite family members? When the conference begins, who will review the ground rules and who will lead the meeting?
- Will the patient participate in the conference? If not, why? Who is the decision maker if the patient does not have capacity?

Decision Making with Families when the Patient Is Unable to Participate
Although many people feel it is optimal to involve patients in all family conferences, the reality is that a large proportion of patients lack decision-making capacity at the end of life, leaving decisions to the family and physicians.[232-234] Complicating this reality is the fact that most

patients do not have advance directives,[235] which, although not always followed perfectly,[236] can provide some direction.[237]

Several excellent guidelines have been published on how to conduct a family meeting and make decisions when patients are unable to participate.[238-241] Many of the communication techniques described here are essential to navigating the decision-making process with families, but two points deserve further emphasis: substituted judgment and enhanced autonomy.

Substituted Judgment
It is important that the family understand the difference between substituted judgment and "best interests."[239] *Substituted judgment* involves trying to determine what the patient would decide if he were able to participate in the discussion. When one decides what is best for the patient independent of what the patient would say, however, this is considered *best interests*. Most guidelines recommend encouraging the family to use substituted judgment when approaching end-of-life decisions because it can help unite family members with differing agendas, refocus family members on the common purpose (ie, honoring the patient's wishes), and may alleviate family guilt after the patient's death.[238-240] This can be accomplished by asking family members questions such as "What would your mother want if she could speak to us now?" or "Did your father ever express his wishes if this kind of situation happened?" Unfortunately surrogates are rarely skilled at predicting patient wishes[242] and struggle with the perceived burden of decision making, especially if they have not had a thoughtful advance care planning discussion with the patient and a clinician.[101,243]

Enhanced Autonomy
Quill and Brody proposed the idea of enhanced autonomy,[181] which has since been incorporated into many guides for decision making at the end of life.[45,238-240] The basic idea, as it has been applied to family meetings, is that the physician should actively explore patient and family values and goals and then integrate this information with the medical facts to offer a clear recommendation for the course of care that would best achieve these goals.[240] This idea has the potential to take some of the decision-making burden off the family and prevent members from feeling as though they're "pulling the plug." Offering these types of value-centered recommendations has been associated with increased satisfaction,[244] but some families do not want recommendations from their physician.[245] The only way to know how families want to make decisions is to ask.[246] Discordance between preferred and actual decision-making roles is associated with higher rates of depression and posttraumatic stress disorder.[247] Most families, however, prefer a shared decision-making model and want to hear the physician's recommendation.[248,249] Many clinicians take the approach of offering rather than imposing recommendations.[250] A sample phrasing may be "Would it be helpful if I gave you my recommendation for what we should do based on where we are medically and what you have told me about your father's wishes?" See the section Achieving a Shared Decision on page 53 and Table 15.

The Medical Decision Maker

Always remember to look for any legal documentation that might designate a medical decision maker, such as a healthcare power of attorney document or a medical living will. If none exists, consult your state's surrogate decision making act or your ethics department for guidance.

Sometimes family members or friends will challenge the decision-making process, or feel slighted by the need to identify the legal next of kin. In such situations, consider saying the following: "We absolutely respect your role in Mr. Smith's life and will certainly turn to you to help get to know him better. We want to make sure we are respecting his wishes every step of the way. In keeping with this goal, we need to identify his legal next of kin to make sure everyone who needs to be involved is able to be involved. I can imagine this might be uncomfortable for some in the family, and we appreciate everyone's patience and understanding."

Roadmaps for Family Conferences

Significant planning may be necessary prior to starting a family meeting. It is important to make sure that all family members who want to be present are there and that you extend invitations to important members of the team such as the primary care physician, chaplain, social worker, and nurse.

Reviewing the medical record in detail and discussing anticipated issues like prognosis, next steps, and treatment options with appropriate consultants often is helpful. Find a quiet room with enough seating and tissues available, and meet with the medical team before going into the family conference to "prebrief" and discuss strategies and goals and personal emotions that might surround the case. Many of the communication techniques used in having a family meeting are discussed elsewhere in this book. The SPIKES protocol for communicating serious news can be easily adapted and used as a roadmap for facilitating a family meeting.[152] See Table 8 for further description.

Another useful tool in assessing goals and focusing on shared decision making in a family meeting is the REMAP technique, which is summarized in Table 14.[179]

Specific Communication and Counseling Techniques

When physicians work with patients and families, their primary responsibility is to perform certain tasks with empathy and careful attention to detail. Helping patients and families understand the suspected diagnosis and prognosis and make sense of what is happening to them are key counseling elements in the physician-patient relationship. It is also important to use empathy when presenting and explaining a suggested medical treatment plan, negotiating with the patient and family until a mutually acceptable plan is established,[251] working with a team to develop an interdisciplinary treatment plan, and providing ongoing guidance and emotional support.

Most patients who have a terminal illness and their family members are not looking for prolonged or formal psychotherapy from their physicians. Instead they want information and guidance so they can make sense of what is happening. They also want support as they search for a renewed sense of purpose, meaning, value, and hope. **Table 19** lists basic communication and counseling techniques that physicians can use during family conferences to elicit the patient and family's concerns and provide appropriate support. Although a physician's first priority is to provide medical attention to the patient, it is important to maintain equal loyalty to all members of the family during these conferences.[122]

Table 19. Communication and Counseling Techniques for Physicians During Family Conferences

Use listening techniques and nonverbal behaviors that communicate empathy and interest, encourage patients and family members to talk, indicate that the physician is listening, and enhance the patient and family's sense of being heard. (See Strategies for Effective Communication on pages 19-27.)

Demystify and correct misconceptions, such as "The use of morphine causes addiction" or "When artificial nutrition is withheld, terminally ill patients suffer and their lives are shortened." (See *UNIPAC 3, UNIPAC 4,* and *UNIPAC 6*). Consider saying, "I hear that you are worried about morphine causing addiction. A lot of people feel the same way. Would it be okay if I explained how I see things and how I would plan to use the medication?"

Acknowledge the family's fear, grief, and guilt; for example, "If only I had fed him more, he wouldn't be so thin" or "If only I had taken her to a different doctor, she wouldn't be dying now." One way to respond is by reframing the situation. For example, "I sense you are feeling a little guilty about not feeding him. I worry that his being so thin is because of his cancer, and he was eating what his body would allow him to eat. I worry that eating more may have actually made him more uncomfortable at this point."

Exhibit equal loyalty to all members of the family, and refrain from taking sides with one or more family members.[1]

Help patients and family members identify their strengths and set realistic short-term goals.

Use reframing to help patients and families recognize other perspectives. For example, "What do you think he would say if he could speak to us now?"

Refocus family members on the common purpose; for example, "We're not asking you to make this decision, but help us understand what your dad would decide so we can honor and respect his wishes."

Help patients and families make sense of what is happening to them by engaging them in an ongoing search for meaning (see *UNIPAC 2*).

On occasion, physicians encounter patients and family members with deep-seated problems for which solutions clearly exceed the physician's skills. It is appropriate in these situations to request the involvement of team members with specialized counseling skills or to consult with team members about referrals to outside sources for specialized counseling or psychiatric treatment.

"Am I starving him?"

Often a major concern for families is the loss of appetite at the end of life, and decisions to not pursue or continue aggressive nutritional support may be very tough to consider. How do you respond to the question "Am I starving him?"

When a patient is at the end of life, one possible statement you can make is "I absolutely hear what you are saying. I can't imagine how distressing it must be thinking about your loved one not eating. At this point his body is shutting down, and I don't think he will feel any hunger. In fact, his body doesn't need food like you or I would need food, and it wouldn't know what to do with all the nutrition. I worry that feeding through a tube at this point would just cause more discomfort, like swelling in his hands and feet."

Anticipating and Mediating Conflict

Patients and family members may differ in their expectations of hospice and palliative care and the goals of treatment, and this may lead to conflict. Forty-six percent of families reported conflict surrounding the cessation of their loved one's life support, and 33% said the conflict was about communication.[252,253] Aggressive attempts to intervene with families at risk for conflict have led to improved decision making.[254] Effective mediation helps resolve conflicts because it

- increases the participants' sense of being heard and clarifies their views and attitudes
- reduces defensiveness and exaggerated positions and statements
- identifies short- and long-term goals
- evaluates as many solutions as possible, emphasizing those that preserve each party's dignity and self-esteem
- encourages participants to identify one solution, which they agree to try and to evaluate
- refocuses attention on the common purpose—what the patient would say in this situation.

One common source of conflict at the end of life is the patient or family who wants "everything" done, as is the case with some of Juanita's family members (see the Clinical Situation on pages 65-66). The usual response when working with patients near the end of life is to try to convince the family that doing everything may not be appropriate. A more effective strategy is to explore what is meant by "everything." Only through clarification of

Communication and Teamwork | 75

families' philosophies regarding end-of-life care can physicians make recommendations for how to best structure interventions to meet their goals. Clarification also allows clinicians to help alleviate moral distress among members of the care team by explaining the patient or family's reasoning and finding shared goals, such as pain control, toward which everyone can work.[255]

Another common source of conflict involves differing opinions regarding religion and spirituality, especially when faith-based belief systems clash with the medical team's perception of reality.[256,257] Offering support from the pastoral care service or community spiritual leaders often is helpful, and exploring issues of faith in family conferences can further clarify goals and expectations. **Table 20** offers some suggestions for exploring faith in a family conference.

Negotiation Strategies to Resolve Conflict

Physicians can use several negotiation strategies to resolve conflicts, including the following[258]:
- Focus on the problem, not the person or personality.
- Clarify the problem.
- Brainstorm possible solutions.
- Focus on common interests.
- Use objective criteria when possible.
- Develop solutions that honor both parties.

The communication techniques discussed earlier in this chapter, including active listening, self-disclosure, giving information clearly, and empathizing, are all especially valuable in these situations.[8,259]

Table 20. Exploring Faith in a Family Conference

Patient/Family Member	Clinician
"I'm praying for a miracle."	"What would a miracle look like?"
	"Is there anything else you are praying for?"
	"What would your father say if God does not grant a miracle?"
"He's very religious. He's a man of God."	"Tell me more about the role faith plays in his life."
	"I can see that faith is a very important part of his life. Has his faith played a role in other medical decisions, either for himself or loved ones?"
"Everything is in God's hands."	"I can see you draw a lot of strength from your faith."
	"Have there been moments when your faith has been tested?"

One proposed framework for understanding conflict involves seeing the conversation as having three levels: facts, emotions, and identity.[98] The goal is not to convince the other side that you are correct but to try to have both sides develop a shared understanding of the relevant facts, each side's emotions, and how the issue influences each side's perception of their identity. After these issues are on the table, finding a common goal becomes much easier.

It is important to remember that effective mediation can improve the negotiation process, but it may not resolve underlying, deep-seated conflicts. When patients are admitted to hospice and palliative care programs, their prognosis is usually limited. Physicians need to acknowledge that some family conflicts can be resolved in the time allotted, but others cannot. When deep-seated conflicts exist, physicians should focus on accomplishing as much as possible and doing as little harm as possible.[260] Sometimes, in the midst of particularly difficult negotiations, a therapeutic technique is to leave the room, notice areas of bodily tension, and breathe deeply until some perspective is regained before reentering the fray. Then, suggest that negotiations resume after everyone has had some time to rethink the issues and can suggest possible solutions.

When Enough Is Enough

Sometimes emotions escalate so dramatically, and conflict is so heated, that little progress can be made in a family meeting. Knowing when to stop pushing and when to regroup at a later time is a valuable skill. If you find that things have reached an impasse, consider the following: "I sense things are quite tense right now, and emotions are running high. I'm worried we won't be able to have an effective conversation right now, which is okay. Perhaps we can regroup in a couple of hours and talk a little more?"

Clinical Situation

Juanita's Case Concludes (continued from page 66)

After discussing Juanita's case with her oncologist, Dr. Owens, and social worker, Mary, Dr. Owens would be willing to offer another course of a different type of palliative chemotherapy but is very concerned about the potential toxicity and effect on quality of life. Mary mentions that Juanita and her family are in one of the larger patient rooms, there is enough seating, and there are tissues on the table. You've clarified with the oncologist that you will lead the meeting, Dr. Owens will provide the clinical updates, and Mary will offer support and guidance and address any social issues that might arise. You enter the room. Juanita is seated. Beside her are her three children, Boni, Juan, and Niki. Her husband, Al, is standing in the corner of the room, notepad in hand. You make introductions and have a seat. Almost immediately her children start talking.

The Conversation	Specific Strategies and Skills
Juan: We definitely want to do everything possible. Mom's a fighter—we want to do whatever you have to offer.	
You: Tell me more about what you mean by "everything."	Exploring with empathy
Juan: Treatment. Chemotherapy, anything to get rid of the cancer.	
You: I see. Thank you for clarifying. We will definitely talk about options moving forward. Before we do, it would be helpful for me if you could tell me what you understand is going on.	Gauging perception (SPIKES)
Juanita: I know I have pancreatic cancer, and it's quite bad. It has spread to my liver and my lungs. I know there will be no cure for it.	Perception matches that of medical team.
Niki: Yeah, but at least we can slow it down, right? Buy some time? That's what this chemo will do, right?	
You: Would it be helpful if Dr. Owens, the oncologist, goes over the treatment options and some of the things we are concerned about?	Asking permission/invitation (SPIKES) Warning shot
Juanita: Yes.	
Dr. Owens: You're right. Your cancer is stage IV. There is no cure, and pancreatic cancer can be quite aggressive. We do have another type of palliative chemotherapy that we can try, but I am worried that the side effects will be quite severe.	Providing knowledge (SPIKES).
Al: Are you saying we shouldn't do it?	Emotional cue? Anger? Disbelief?
Dr. Owens: No, but I think we should really think about how it will affect the quality of the time you have left.	
Juanita: How much…time do I have?	
Dr. Owens: I'm worried that without treatment you may have less than 6 months. With treatment, maybe only a few months more.	Providing prognosis/knowledge, reframing expectations of prognosis (REMAP)
Juanita *(crying)*: Six months?	Emotional cue: shock, disbelief

You: *(Silence)* You weren't expecting to hear that.	Responding to emotional cue with empathy (REMAP, SPIKES).
Juanita: No. I thought I'd have more time than 6 months.	
Niki: Yeah, but isn't there something we can do to get more time? Experimental trials?	
You: I really wish there was.	"I wish" statement.
Juanita: So it's less than a year.	
You: *(Silence)* Looking ahead, what are some of the things that are important to you?	Using silence
	Assessing the patient's values, mapping the future (REMAP).
Juanita: My…my family, being with my family. And not suffering.	Patient's goals and values.
Juan: But you can't give up, Mom. You're going to be a grandmother. We need you to be there.	Emotional cue: fear of abandonment?
Al: We have to try something. Something's better than nothing at all.	
Mary: I can't imagine how hard it is to think about this. You are all doing such a great job thinking about what Juanita values, while balancing your own hopes.	Responding to emotions with empathy, refocusing on the common purpose
Boni: We all just want her to get better.	Refocused on common purpose: Juanita's health
You: I think that's a wonderful and loving thing to hope for. Is there anything else you are all hoping for?	Providing support, respect statement
	Exploring hope
Juanita: More time.	

? Is there anything you would have said or done differently?

? How would you react to a request to "do everything"?

? How do you provide feedback to a colleague? Is there any feedback you would give to the oncologist?

? How do you process a plan of care that you might not personally agree with? Do you have your own coping strategies?

Selected Communication Issues

Clinical Situation

Charles

You are a hospice chaplain on an inpatient unit. Charles, a 50-year-old patient with lung cancer, is experiencing unrelieved pain, breathlessness, and restlessness. During a visit with you, Charles indicates he is extremely fearful of dying and wants to confide a secret. After being assured of the chaplain's respect for confidentiality, Charles relates that while serving in Vietnam he murdered several civilians and had a child out of wedlock. Now he is fearful of eternal retribution and is consumed with guilt for the indiscriminate killings, abandoning the child and mother, and keeping the child a secret from his wife, Vickie.

You know that, in addition to Charles, other people are suffering as the result of Charles's psychological and spiritual distress. The team physician has been treating Charles's restlessness, pain, and dyspnea with increasing dosages of medication without success and is now questioning her competence. The social worker is deeply concerned about Charles's obvious but unvoiced emotional distress and is questioning his inability to effectively intervene. Vickie is experiencing an increased sense of isolation from her husband; she wants to comfort Charles but senses that, once again, he is shutting her out.

- Which details, if any, regarding Charles's fears of dying and worries about prior events should you share with the interdisciplinary team?

- How can you respect Charles' confidentiality while still supporting the team in their work and perhaps provide additional comfort to Charles?

- Can you share confidential information if it directly benefits the patient?

Case continues on page 82

Confidentiality

In hospice and palliative care settings, patients retain the right to confidentiality.[261] When dying patients and their family members entrust healthcare professionals with their fears, anxieties, regrets, and unfulfilled dreams, they are likely to assume the information will remain confidential.[262]

Confidentiality is not an absolute obligation. Information can be revealed if the patient's condition poses a risk to others, but it must be highly valued.[263] In some cases, concerns arise when a patient shares confidential information with one team member about past events that are causing psychological or spiritual pain and interfering with the management of physical symptoms in the present. For example, when anxiety, guilt, fear, remorse, or sadness exacerbate physical symptoms that are being treated unsuccessfully with increased dosages of medications, the team member is likely to struggle with the issue of how much to tell and to whom.

In most cases, patients are willing to negotiate the amount of information shared so their right to privacy is protected without compromising the team's ability to effectively intervene. Confidentiality is breached when the patient believes information shared with one team member will be kept confidential but is shared with other team members without the patient's authorization. Hospice and palliative care programs should develop policies about patient confidentiality and the sharing of sensitive information. If a patient does not want specific information shared with the rest of the team, balancing the patient's right to privacy with the team's need for information can present ethical dilemmas, particularly when continued secrecy may result in inappropriate treatments.[68]

Clinical Situation

Charles's Case Concludes (continued from page 81)

During the course of several conversations over the next few days, the chaplain reassures Charles that he is a valued and loved human being despite his past failings. The chaplain reminds Charles that other people care about him, and he tries to negotiate with Charles to share some information so the team can intervene more effectively. Charles agrees to let the chaplain share information about his situation, but only with the physician and only if the actual deeds are not divulged. The chaplain agrees. During the next several weeks, the chaplain encourages Charles to express his love to Vickie. The chaplain also continues to support Charles's search for ways to come to terms with his entire life.

Communication with Colleagues and Referring Providers

Much of modern palliative medicine is practiced in the role of consultant, most commonly via inpatient palliative care consultation services. These consultations occur not only in inpatient units but increasingly in other settings such as emergency departments (EDs) and intensive care units (ICUs). Trials of palliative care consultation in the ICU have shown mixed results, with positive studies generally encompassing the entire team, including the physician.[264-267] There is less research and fewer solid positive outcomes in the ED,[265] but the ED has been identified as a place that hosts common palliative care issues[268,269] in which palliative care principles can influence care,[270] especially if provided by the whole team.[271,272] Independent of the setting, however, communication issues are often the barrier to more successful consultations.[273,274] In recent years there has been a surge of interest in developing triggers for palliative care consultation, although there are numerous logistical challenges, such as short hospital stays, provider resistance, and high acuity of symptoms.[275] Consultation screening tools are also being developed, with one recent study showing increased palliative care consultation with the use of a seven-point screening tool for medical ICU patients.[276]

Regardless of setting, if a palliative care consultation service is to be effective, the consultant must understand how appropriate etiquette frames communication with patients, families, and consulting teams.[277] Although many of the issues for palliative care consult services are the same as for any consult service,[278,279] the main struggle for palliative care clinicians is to balance being a patient advocate and being a good consultant who does not undermine the referring clinician. The key to successfully navigating this road is to address only the consult question with the patient. Any other concerns that arise during the consultation should be negotiated with the primary team before discussing them with the patient. If the patient brings up other concerns, they should be heard, but no plans should be enacted and no new information disclosed without first talking to the team. This does not mean the palliative care physician should abandon the patient and her needs, only that addressing these needs should happen after getting buy-in from the doctors in charge of the patient's care. Although this sounds simple, these discussions can be difficult because they often involve challenging the primary physician's management plan. Humility is essential to making these conversations work. The palliative care clinician's approach should be to acknowledge that the primary team may know things about the patient that the palliative care team does not know and to assume they are well-meaning, intelligent physicians. The goal of the discussion should be to understand what the primary team physicians know and why they are approaching the patient's care in this manner.[231] Using this approach, a negotiation about how to work together to best meet the patient's needs is much more likely to succeed. In the case of Ethel (see the Clinical Situation on page 61), the team's request may simply reflect its interactions with the family, and family members may be open to exploring their concerns with you and trying an "informed refusal" strategy.

As consultants, palliative care providers generally work with patients and families at the request of another physician. Many physicians who care for dying patients (eg, in the ICU, ED, and during oncology visits) will admit that communicating with patients and families is the most stressful part of their job[280] and that palliative care and hospice physicians and staff are experts at conducting difficult conversations with patients and families. Yet physicians may be resistant to consult a hospice or palliative medicine team because of the perceived implication of "giving up." Modeling communication behaviors similar to those used with patients is the most successful approach to interacting with colleagues in difficult situations.

It is vital that consultants respect the relationship between themselves and the responsible physician requesting advice and the relationships between the physician and the patient and family.[281] If the hospice and palliative medicine consultant is careful to honor those relationships, the relationship with the referring physician will be preserved, and it is much more likely that the consultant will be asked to see many additional patients in the future. Caring for relationships with colleagues will allow consultants to interact with many more patients over time.

Table 21 outlines an approach that mirrors the shared decision-making process for instances when a colleague calls for a consultation.

Communication with Patients with Dementia and Their Caregivers

Communication with patients with dementia and their caregivers can be guided by many of the principles already discussed in Facilitating Family Conferences (see page 71). There are, however, some unique considerations (see *UNIPAC 9*).

Physicians may be challenged with the following communication tasks,[282] which unfortunately are often performed ineffectively:[283]

- explaining the diagnosis, prognosis, and disease progression
- preparing for a lack of decision-making capacity by creating an advance directive and naming a proxy, if possible
- explaining safety issues such as not driving
- assisting in the transition to a nursing home, if necessary, which may include providing emotional support to the family upon transfer to avoid feelings of having failed the patient.

Physicians are also responsible for educating patients with dementia and their families about nutrition and hydration. Many families struggle as the patient's oral intake declines. Normalizing this change as part of the natural progression of the disease and encouraging oral feedings as tolerated is usually the best approach.[284] More than 85% of patients with advanced dementia develop eating problems,[285] and feeding tubes do not appear to provide benefit and are not recommended for people with advanced dementia.[286] Like nutrition, hydration can be a struggle for families. Again, it is usually best to normalize this change as part of the disease and reassure the caregivers the patient will take what he needs and that the only symptomatic concern is usually a dry mouth.[284]

Pneumonia is the most common cause of death for patients with advanced dementia.[287] Even if antibiotics prolong life in the late stages, they may worsen discomfort.[288] It is incumbent on the physician to explain this to the family and ensure excellent symptom control with antipyretics and analgesics.

Families will often grieve each time the patient experiences a decline in function. Helping the family during the grieving process is of primary importance. There also may be a sense of detachment that occurs as the patient's disease progresses. There may even be a wish for the patient's death, which should be normalized as a wish for relief from suffering. Support groups and a focus on relieving a sense of guilt may be helpful.[289] Sometimes the introduction of hospice care may reignite the grieving process as the patient's imminent death becomes more real to the family, but research has shown that families of patients with dementia who received hospice care have fewer concerns about unmet needs and quality of care.[290] Because primary

Table 21. A Method for Optimizing Communication Between the Hospice and Palliative Medicine Consultant and a Consulting Physician

Model	Context	Suggested Phrases
Orientation		
Define the problem	Ask enough questions to be certain you understand the problem.	"How can I help?"
		"Can you tell me more about why the family is difficult?"
		"Just to be clear, you want me to focus on his pain and not discuss anything about prognosis."
Set goals	Clarify the physician's hopes for the outcome of your consultation.	"What are you hoping I'll be able to achieve with this family?"
		"So, you're hoping we can decrease his pain by 50% by tomorrow?"
Plan the process	Clarify your expectations (especially if they are different from the consulting physician's) and establish a timetable.	"I think I can help this family come to terms with discontinuing ventilator support, but I suspect it will take several visits with them over a few days."
		"I will come and see them this afternoon and get back to you with my thoughts, okay?"
		"If they happen to bring up end-of-life wishes, then I will explore them as gently as possible, keeping in mind all of your concerns and the current treatment plan."
Discussion		
Gather information	Meet and evaluate the patient.	
Identify potential solutions	Identify and evaluate potential solutions and decide on a course of action.	
Making a Recommendation		
	Make your recommendations both in the medical record and by personal communication, preferably face to face or over the phone.	Use empathetic statements: "Boy, this is a difficult situation." (Pause for response.) "I would suggest…"

Continued on page 86

Table 21. A Method for Optimizing Communication Between the Hospice and Palliative Medicine Consultant and a Consulting Physician (continued)

Model	Context	Suggested Phrases
Implementation		
Adhere to the decision	Follow up with the physician, patient, and family.	"I see your pain medications have been increased. I will see you tomorrow morning to see how this increase worked."
Evaluate the response	Assess the effectiveness of your recommendations and ongoing intervention.	"I saw the patient this morning and it seems his pain is better but still not well controlled. What is your sense of how things are going?"
Seek feedback	Solicit input from the consulting physician, appropriate staff, and patient and family.	"I just want to check in with you about Mr. Smith; any questions or concerns?"
		"It's important that I provide you and your patients with excellent service. Do you have any feedback on things you wish went differently on the Smith case?"

caregivers have taken care of the patient for so long, the hospice team must help them let go of the caregiving experience that has become a part of their lives.[291]

Communicating with a patient with dementia can be difficult, especially as the disease progresses. There are guidelines based on the various stages of patient communication. For example, when a patient is alert and talking but saying something incorrect, the physician does not have to agree with them; however, it is usually better to not try to convince them of reality. Instead, try to go where the patient is by empathizing with the situation and asking questions. If the patient is displaying nonsensical speech, try to mirror their emotions, unless the patient appears anxious. In this case, it is best to speak in a calm tone, avoid sudden movements, and reassure the patient by touching, making direct nonthreatening eye contact, and sitting at eye level or lower. If a patient is no longer speaking, continue to speak in reassuring tones. Hearing familiar voices, music, or prayers can be soothing. Appeal to all senses with familiar smells, gentle touch, and favorite tastes. Try to move and speak slowly so the patient has time to process and is not startled.[291]

In more advanced stages, it is important to watch for nonverbal pain indicators such as a facial grimace, furrowing of the brow, or agitation. Perform pain medication trials to see if they resolve these behaviors (see *UNIPAC 3* and *UNIPAC 9*).[291] Studies have shown that communication skill training in dementia care can improve quality of life and well-being and increase positive interactions with patients and caregivers.[292]

Communicating with Young Children of Dying Patients

Patients with a terminal diagnosis will often ask how to talk with their children about their illness. Children process the death of a parent in different ways at different ages; consequently, a developmentally appropriate strategy is necessary. A complete discussion of how to counsel children with a dying parent is beyond the scope of this book; see *UNIPAC 7* for a discussion about communicating with children and families about palliative care, terminal illness, and death. A social worker on the hospice team with this type of special training can be invaluable, and a child life specialist can provide expert guidance in speaking with children at their developmental levels.[293] However, often these questions are directed to the physician. To address such situations, guidelines about talking with children of certain age groups can be helpful to physicians.[294,295]

Children between 3 and 5 years of age do not always comprehend what it means for their parent to be dying, and they may not understand death as being permanent. They can, however, memorize a script about what is happening; having such a script can be helpful. It can be valuable to find a substitute caregiver and reassure children that they will be taken care of and are loved. Intense expressions of grief can be alarming to children this age, so it is important to prepare children for visits and carefully structure time.

Children between 6 and 8 years of age tend to have a better understanding of death and its permanence, but they may still make logical mistakes and find it difficult to reverse their thinking. Children at this age may blame themselves and can become highly emotional. It is helpful to give them simple, straightforward information about the disease and how it causes symptoms and behaviors. They can be more involved in visits to the hospital, rituals, and bereavement programs. Enlisting other professionals to listen to the child's distress can relieve parents.[296]

Children between 9 and 11 years of age think much more logically and tend to benefit from detailed information given incrementally. Compared with younger children who primarily feel anxiety, children in this age group often experience sadness and loss and often find it valuable to become involved in the patient's care.

Communication with the Dying Patient

Toward the end of the dying process, some terminally ill patients speak in rambling, disjointed phrases that may indicate either delirium or significant final communications. Some authors believe the extraordinary experiences described by dying patients are near-death experiences with special meanings.[297] In their book *Final Gifts,* Callanan and Kelley recommend educating family members about common themes that can help them decipher special meanings in the patient's final communications.[298]

For example, terminally ill patients frequently see or talk to someone who has already died. They also may communicate about going home, standing in line, or going on a trip. These may be references to the patient's desire to complete the dying process—they may want permission to die. Some dying patients glimpse other worlds or feel as if they are in another place. Others may have end-of-life dreams and visions that significantly impact the predeath experience.[299] Usually the dreams or feelings are comforting, but sometimes they create groundless anxieties about mental dysfunction. Some dying patients appear to wait until after they have had a chance to visit with a special family member before dying. On other occasions they may wait until someone has left the room. Very private people may prefer to die when they are alone. Some terminally ill patients appear to know when they are going to die, even when the usual signs of rapidly approaching death are absent. Patients may call a loved one in the morning to say goodbye, seeming to know that death will occur before the next scheduled visit.

These possible phases and states of mind may be important to discuss with family caregivers. Not all patients will experience them, but it is important to be prepared. Throughout the dying process, caregivers should continue to communicate reassurance and support. They can do this by responding in an accepting way to whatever the patient sees or hears, asking gentle questions about what the patient is seeing, and repeating statements that aren't understood. Patients need support during the dying process. It is important to acknowledge their difficulty letting go or understand when they prefer to remain silent.

Families often ask about the meaning of patient movements when they are unresponsive. Although these may be simple cognitive questions, often they are accompanied by strong emotions. Physicians generally respond to such questions with only clinical information,[300] but there may be benefit to attending to the underlying emotion as well. It is usually easy to keep patients comfortable during the last hours of life, and the clinician's real task becomes caring for the family by communicating effectively in this time of great need.

Communication Strategies During Telehealth Encounters

Telemedicine is the use of medical information exchanged from one site to another via electronic communications to improve a patient's clinical health status.[301] A variety of applications and services can be used for connecting patient and provider in this manner, including two-way video, email, and phone. The use of telemedicine is becoming more common[301] and is becoming a valuable resource for providing palliative care. Several successful models that use telemedicine have been described in the literature and include teleconsultation and family meeting by a tertiary care center ICU for patients in rural hospitals being considered for transfer,[302] Web conferencing with outpatients for palliative care symptom management,[303,304] short message service (SMS) text messaging between physicians and patients for outpatient pain medication management, and phone-based interventions to monitor symptoms and provide advice.[305] Although concerns have been raised that the remote nature of telemedicine will hinder the patient-physician relationship,[306] telemedicine often provides access to palliative care services that would otherwise be unavailable. By applying the essential elements of effective communication described below, barriers to face-to-face communication can be minimized.

During a telemedicine encounter, because the physician and patient are not located within physical proximity, it is reasonable to assume that the dynamics will differ slightly from a traditional face-to-face encounter. Although many approaches used in face-to-face encounters remain essential for effective communication in a telemedicine encounter (see Strategies for Effective Communication on pages 19-27), additional strategies and skills need to be considered (**Table 22**).

Table 22. Tips for Effective Telemedicine Communication

Video-Based Technology[307]

Ensure participants do not have hearing or visual impairments.

Ensure audio/video components are working before initiating consultation.

Position the webcam as close as possible to the projected image of the patient so it appears you are making eye contact with the patient.

Minimize distractions and maintain eye contact with the patient.

Use the camera zoom feature to closely monitor patient nonverbal communication.

Compassionate silence may feel awkward. Verbal statements of empathy and compassion are likely to be more effective.[8]

Text-Based Technology

Ensure participants are literate and without vision impairments.

Use clear, concise wording and statements, avoiding medical jargon.

Write at a fifth grade or lower reading level.

Avoid sarcasm and euphemisms that can be taken out of context without nonverbal cues.

Use spell check.

Phone-Based Technology

Ensure clear phone connection and minimize background noises.

Ensure participants do not have hearing impairments.

Make note of all participants at the beginning of the encounter through introductions.

If there are many participants involved in the conversation, it can be helpful to have each individual identify themselves when speaking.

Avoid sarcasm and euphemisms that can be taken out of context without nonverbal cues.

Compassionate silence may feel awkward. Verbal statements of empathy and compassion are likely to be more effective.[8]

Limited English Proficiency

As described in the Limited English Proficiency section (page 17), a significant portion of the US population identifies as speaking English less than "very well," placing them at risk for impaired patient-physician communication.[308] For a variety of reasons (time constraints, lack of access, reimbursement issues), physicians often may feel that it's easier to rely on the patient's family, friends, and neighbors for interpretation. Physicians need to realize that using nonprofessional interpreters can result in distorted information. This can lead to problems such as undermining patient confidentiality, embarrassing and inhibiting patients, exposing children to sensitive information, subverting family dynamics, and providing incomplete information, all of which can result in incomplete histories, ineffective treatments, and inadequate follow-up. Distractions also may limit patients' disclosure of psychosocial and spiritual concerns.[308,309]

Physicians can improve communication by using professional medical interpreters.[309] It is important to differentiate interpreters from translators. *Interpreters* work with spoken words, whereas *translators* work with written words. It also is important to differentiate interpreters from those who are multilingual—being fluent alone does not make one an effective interpreter.[308] Professional interpreters are subject to specific training and credentialing to ensure competence.[309] When live professional medical interpreters are not available, phone interpretation services or Web-based videoconferencing platforms can be used.

Even when using professional interpreters, obstacles remain to achieving effective communication, especially at the end of life. A survey of professional interpreters found that while most felt comfortable participating in end-of-life discussions, only half felt these conversations went well, citing deficits in cultural sensitivity, establishing trust, and general communication skills. Communication can be improved by clearly defining the role of the interpreter and the objectives of the meeting prior to engaging with the patient.[309] Additional tips for optimizing communication via an interpreter are listed in **Table 23**.[308]

Communication with Patients Who Are Lesbian, Gay, Bisexual, and Transgender

The goal of effective, genuine communication in any area of life is to transcend labels and connect with the unique and individual human being on the other side of your sentence. The communication skills discussed in this book strive to build a communication style that is nonjudgmental and supportive regardless of belief or bias. The abbreviation *LGBT* (lesbian, gay, bisexual, transgender) often is used to broadly label the complex psychosocial and health needs of a larger nonheterosexual population. It is estimated that by 2050 LGBT individuals older than 65 years will account for 1 of every 13 older adults in the United States.[310] Mindful and respectful communication customized to an individual's unique experience is key.

One thing to bear in mind is that individuals who identify as LGBT often have nontraditional definitions of family, often encompassing friends rather than biological family members. Social

Table 23. Tips for Using an Interpreter

Identify patients who may need an interpreter.

Allow extra time for the interview.

Meet with the interpreter before the interview to give some background, build rapport, and set goals.

Document the name of the interpreter in the progress note.

Realize that most patients understand some English, so do not make comments you do not want them to understand.

Seat the interpreter next to or slightly behind the patient.

Speak directly to the patient, not the interpreter.

Use first-person statements ("I" statements); avoid saying "he said" or "tell her."

Speak in short sentences or short thought groups.

Ask only one question at a time.

Allow appropriate time for the interpreter to finish the statement.

Prioritize and limit the key points to three or fewer.

Do not use idioms, acronyms, jargon, or humor.

Insist on sentence-by-sentence interpretation to avoid tangential conversations.

Allow 10-minute breaks for every hour of interpretation.

Use the "teach back" or "show me" technique to ensure patient comprehension.

Have a postsession discussion with the interpreter to get further details and make corrections, if necessary.

From "Appropriate Use of Medical Interpreters" (Table 1), by Juckett G, Unger K, Am Fam Physician, *2014;90(7):476-480. © 2014 American Academy of Family Physicians. Reproduced with permission.*[308]

support groups often play larger roles, and surrogate decision making may be affected by conflicts between individual definitions of family and legal definitions. Inquiring about a person's support system and definition of family is important. Terms such as "husband" or "wife" may confine an individual to a set of assumptions or preconceptions, whereas terms such as "life partner" or "significant other" are more encompassing.[311] In addition, past experiences with the healthcare system may affect a person's willingness to communicate about sexuality. Empathetic communications skills such as naming and the use of respect statements are helpful.

Examples of exploratory questions include "Who do you consider family?" and "Tell me more about your support system." Examples of respectful and supportive statements include "Thank you for sharing your experience with me," "We will be here with you every step of the way. Are there specific support groups that you have turned to in the past?" and "Is there anything else you feel I should know to better support you and your loved ones?" **Table 24** and **Table 25** provide further examples of communication techniques and specific palliative care considerations and needs of patients who identify as LGBT.[311]

Table 24. Communication with Nonheterosexual Individuals

Explore sexual orientation	"What do I need to know about you as a person to provide the best care possible?"
Acknowledge identity • Avoid assumptions about identity • Reflect the terms/pronouns used by the patient	"How do you self-identify?" "Am I am using the term or pronoun that you prefer?"
Identify family of choice • Avoid assumptions about who patient considers family • Reflect the terms used by the patient to identify significant relationships	Terms like "partner" or "significant other" may be preferred over "husband" or "wife." "Who do you consider family?" "Are you currently in an intimate relationship?"
Create a welcoming environment	Accept patient's views, feelings, and preferences without judgment. Acknowledge potential discrimination in staff. Empathize with current and past hardships. Provide support and describe a partnership between patient and physician. Consider nonverbal visibility strategies for healthcare spaces such as local or regional visual signs designed to convey respect for all people.

From "Lesbian, Gay, Bisexual, and Transgender Communication" (Chapter 28), by Candrian C, Lum H. In: Wittenberg E, Ferrell BR, Goldsmith J, Smith T, Glajchen M, Handzo GF, eds., Textbook of Palliative Care Communication, *Oxford University Press, 2015. © 2015 Oxford University Press. Reproduced with permission.*[311]

Table 25. Palliative Care Needs of Nonheterosexual Individuals

Health Disparities Related to Serious Illness
- Higher rates of certain cancers/chronic illness
- Higher rates of HIV
- Higher rates of mental health issues

Advance Care Planning and Advance Directives
- Completion of documents so preferences for end-of-life care are honored
- Completion of documents so preferences for surrogate decision makers are honored, especially for same sex partner
- Communicating preferences and choices for end-of-life care to biological family

Family Involvement and Support
- Identifying who patient considers "family"; may include same-sex partner and friends other than biological family
- May have strained relationships with biological family
- Lack of LGBT cancer and chronic illness support groups

End-of-Life Care and Closure
- Potential experiences of victimization and discrimination during life that may necessitate counseling
- Reunion and reconciliation with estranged family and friends that may incite complex dynamic between family of choice and biological family
- Lack of reunion and reconciliation may incite feelings of grief, loss, abandonment
- Disenfranchised grief for partner and family of choice

From "Lesbian, Gay, Bisexual, and Transgender Communication" (Chapter 28), by Candrian C, Lum H. In: Wittenberg E, Ferrell BR, Goldsmith J, Smith T, Glajchen M, Handzo GF, eds., Textbook of Palliative Care Communication, Oxford University Press, 2015. © 2015 Oxford University Press. Reproduced with permission.[311]

Communication Surrounding Organ Donation

Conversations about organ donation near the end of life are a necessary yet understandably challenging issue. In the United States solid organ donation is the most common type[312] involving a variety of organs including the heart, lung, liver, kidney, and pancreas. Organ donation and procurement is strictly regulated and guided by firm ethical principles, and the conversations regarding organ donation are beyond the scope of palliative communication skills. For these reasons, 58 federally designated not-for-profit organ procurement organizations (OPOs) have been created to help facilitate the safe and ethical procurement of organs for transplantation, coordinate the donation process when donors become available, and increase the number of registered donors through community outreach programs and education. Examples of federally designated OPOs include the Center for Organ Recovery and Education and the New England Organ Bank.

While communication with patients and families regarding organ donation is often limited to representatives from a designated OPO, communication by the palliative care team often involves planning and preparation for the end of life, symptom control, and emotional support.[313] The palliative care team's role involves identifying appropriate medical decision makers, living wills, and advance directives; confirming goals and values; and honoring and respecting end-of-life wishes.[314] Decisions to discontinue life-sustaining therapies using the empathetic communication techniques previously discussed is a key role of the palliative care team. After this decision has been made, a representative of the OPO will meet with the family to discuss specifics regarding organ donation and procurement.

Organ Donation

Before cessation of life-sustaining therapy, make sure that a representative from the regional OPO has been contacted to discuss organ donation with the patient and/or family. The palliative care team is not expected to have this conversation.

Simply let the family know that "another member of the team will stop by to speak with you more about some additional next steps and things to expect."

The Interdisciplinary Team

Teamwork represents a set of values that encourage[s] listening and constructive response to the views expressed by others, giving others the benefit of the doubt, providing support, and recognizing the interests and achievements of others. Such values help teams perform, and they also promote individual performance as well as the performance of an entire organization.[315]

—Jon Katzenbach and Douglas Smith

If they don't have scars, they haven't worked on a team. Teams don't just happen. They slowly and painfully evolve. The process is never complete. The work involved is usually underestimated.[316]

—Balfour Mount, MD

Suffering and the Interdisciplinary Team Approach to Care

Profound illness is associated with a sense of loss affecting all aspects of life.[317] Significant losses may upset a person's entire sense of self. When an individual's loss is sufficiently injurious, it causes suffering, which Cassell defines as "a state of severe distress associated with events that threaten the intactness of the person."[317] According to Cassell, "suffering continues until the threat of disintegration has passed or until the integrity of the person can be restored in some other manner."[317]

Because hospice and palliative care practitioners focus on alleviating all aspects of suffering—physical, emotional, and spiritual—for patients and their family members, comprehensive care of terminally ill patients requires the skills and resources of a multidisciplinary team of healthcare professionals.[318] The combined perspectives of interdisciplinary team (IDT) members are much more likely to meet the complex needs of dying patients and their families than any individual provider. Team support can also help physicians cope with their own suffering and grief.

Clinical Situation

Dr. Claiborne

Dr. Claiborne is a 40-year-old family practice physician who has served as the part-time medical director of a community hospice and palliative care program for 2 years. He enjoys working as a member of an interdisciplinary team (IDT) and feels the program provides good symptom control and emotional support for patients and family members.

During the past year and a half, the hospice and palliative care program's daily census gradually expanded to approximately 90 patients. At the same time, recent changes in reimbursement have substantially reduced the operating budget, resulting in the layoff of several long-standing staff members. Dr. Claiborne particularly misses one of the nurses and a social worker, both of whom he valued immensely as sources of information and good patient care. He feels the program's quality of care is suffering. His growing concern about the program is affecting his relationship with the program's administrator.

> **?** How does task-related conflict, such as disagreement about patient care loads, influence team performance?

> **?** What are some routine team processes that can help to identify and manage conflict on the team?

> **?** How does dependence on a single team member for a function influence the function of the team as a whole?

The Function of the Team

The primary goal of a hospice and palliative care IDT is to identify patient and family suffering. Each member of the team represents a particular discipline and approaches problems from a unique perspective. Ideally team members share their individual assessments to create a comprehensive understanding of the issues a patient and family must face. The comprehensive assessment allows the team to develop a multifaceted plan of care that addresses the complex needs of each patient and family. The plan should respect the values, beliefs, and goals of individual patients and their families. Although healthcare professionals recommend interventions, patients and families implement them.

Dying patients' clinical status changes frequently, often deleteriously. The IDT must be capable of rapidly adapting to changes in a patient's condition. The IDT approach to care, while labor intensive, is more likely to address the myriad causes of suffering than attempts made by individual providers. The following mnemonic describes the process of developing a plan of care for patients:

- **P** Perform a thorough review of the patient's history and life story that addresses all the contributors to symptoms and suffering (eg, physical, emotional, social, spiritual). Listen carefully to life stories told by patients and family members.
- **L** Look at objective data. Obtain necessary information from the medical record, history and physical examination, and self-assessment scales (which may measure physical pain, depression, or quality of life); consider the need for laboratory work, imaging, or other information.
- **A** Assess information. Assess all information provided by patients, family members, team members, laboratory tests, and self-assessment scales.
- **N** Negotiate the treatment plan. Develop an individualized patient care plan with other members of the team. Consider the patient's values, beliefs, and goals. Negotiate the plan with the patient and family. Revise the plan as needed to better meet the patient's and family's values, beliefs, goals, and changing clinical status.

Requirements for a Hospice IDT

In the United States the IDT approach to caring for patients with terminal illness is mandated by the Medicare hospice benefit. Reimbursement depends on a hospice program's ability to meet basic criteria, which include an interdisciplinary team assessment and care plan for each enrolled patient that is updated at least every 15 days. The IDT must include, at minimum, the following core members: a physician, a registered nurse, a social worker, and a pastoral or other counselor.[319] (For more information on the Medicare hospice benefit, see *UNIPAC 1* and AAHPM's *Hospice Medical Director Manual*.[320]) A qualified physician is required to coordinate this team.[321]

Medicare regulations and National Hospice and Palliative Care Organization guidelines recognize some variations in team composition and frequency of team meetings. Medicare requires minimum participation of four core members in team meetings. Medicare also requires that each patient be discussed at an IDT meeting every 2 weeks. Ideally, each patient and family is evaluated separately by core team members before the development of a comprehensive plan of care. The recommendations are negotiated with the patient and family until a mutually agreed-upon plan is devised.

Cost-related concerns affect the frequency and composition of team meetings. Because team meetings do not generate revenue, some programs limit the frequency of these meetings to the Medicare minimum or include only supervisory staff in team meetings. A hospice IDT that meets solely to fulfill Medicare requirements may fall short of its primary function to relieve suffering. In today's financial climate, it is important for team members to communicate effectively, represent their discipline in an assertive manner, and insist that programs meet the physical, emotional, social, and spiritual needs of dying patients and their families.

General Characteristics of the IDT

What Is a Team?

Teams are defined by several key characteristics. Members work to achieve a shared goal, and their behavior and outcomes are interdependent. Team membership ideally is bound and stable over time, and the team operates in a social-system context.[322]

This definition of teams also is a perfect fit for IDTs regardless of setting (ie, hospice IDT versus inpatient consult service IDT). For members of an IDT, the shared goal is to identify and manage suffering among patients and families. The team members are interdependent, meaning they cannot relieve total pain (spiritual, emotional, physical, psychological) unilaterally; they must rely on teamwork. The members of an IDT are generally stable over many months or years, and they meet as a group regularly. The IDT works within the larger context of a patient's social network, which includes the patient, family, friends, and the primary physician. The IDT also works within the broader healthcare system and interacts with the system to benefit its patients. **Table 26** describes an IDT and lists some of its advantages and disadvantages.[323]

Developmental Phases

Like other groups, IDTs undergo a sometimes painful developmental process. When faced with crises such as staff cutbacks, mergers, or the loss of key members, even the most effective teams are likely to experience developmental setbacks.[324,325] **Table 27** describes the observed developmental phases of interdisciplinary healthcare teams.[326]

Table 26. The Interdisciplinary Team: Description, Advantages, and Disadvantages

Description

Involves more than one discipline

Shares information and sets team goals

Is interdependent, with shared responsibility

Is structured to encourage collaboration

Works on team problems

Shifts leadership, depending on specific issues and areas of expertise

Advantages

Integrates many perspectives

Encourages teamwork to craft creative solutions to difficult problems

Develops formal and informal solutions to address complex problems

Develops solutions with depth and breadth

Shares responsibility for leadership

Empowers individuals on the team

Provides a network of support for team members

Disadvantages

Initially, decisions take more time

Members must learn the vocabulary and perspectives of other disciplines

Effort is needed to maintain the team

The team requires time and space to clarify values, renegotiate roles, and resolve conflicts

Individuals require time to develop leadership skills

Building the Team

Characteristics of Effective Teams

In general, effective teams agree on a common set of principles, goals, and measurable objectives.[281,315] Effective teams depend on and expect competent individual members to represent their discipline's current practice standards. Effective teams share the responsibility for team functioning[324] and provide ongoing feedback in team interaction, leadership, communication, and conflict resolution.[327] Hospice and palliative care teams are often large and members frequently change, so a strong culture of enabling members to speak up about the team process is imperative to create and maintain an effective team.

Table 27. Developmental Phases of Interdisciplinary Healthcare Teams

Phase I. Forming

Superficial information, such as name and background, is shared.

Members size each other up and test each other; they categorize each other by outside roles and status.

Members are guarded, more impersonal than personal; a few are active, and others are passive.

Uncertainty over purpose exists.

Conflict is neither discussed nor addressed.

Phase II. Norming

An attempt is made to establish common goals.

The team establishes ground rules and begins to clarify common roles.

Mistrust is exhibited by caution and conformity.

Role overlap becomes evident.

A few members attempt to establish bonds with others who have similar views.

The team may want leader(s) to assume responsibility.

Strategies are used to increase equality of leadership (eg, rotate leadership).

Defensive communication and disruptive behavior increases.

Frustration exists among team members.

Some members project blame and responsibility toward the perceived leaders.

Competition exists among team members.

Some members come to meetings late or do not attend.

Continued on page 100

Table 27. Developmental Phases of Interdisciplinary Healthcare Teams (continued)

Phase III. Confrontation

Conflicts can no longer be avoided, and some members verbally attack other members.

Increased conflicts over leadership, equality, and commitment arise.

Members experience anxiety over expression of affect.

Some conflicts are addressed in a direct manner.

Some members withdraw from the team.

The search begins for leaders who will resolve conflicts.

Functional leaders emerge.

Realization occurs that power is not equal.

Realization occurs that everyone has power for leadership and decision making.

Constructive confrontation results when conflicts occur.

Goals and roles are reclarified.

Coalitions form but change according to team needs.

The following conditions are essential for effective teamwork[328]:
- a clear and elevating goal
- a results-driven structure that emphasizes clear roles and accountability and uses effective communication with performance measures and feedback
- competent team members
- unified commitment
- a collaborative working environment
- normative standards of excellence
- external support and recognition
- internal support of team members and interest in each other's well being
- principled leadership.

Table 28 summarizes the characteristics of effective IDTs.[315,324,327,329-331]

Institutional Support

IDTs require institutional support to be effective. This includes a commitment to hire knowledgeable professionals with strong skills in communication and problem solving who will assertively represent their discipline's unique body of knowledge.[327] Continuing education and training related to professional skills and team functioning is also vital for teams to be effective. Institutions can provide organizational resources, such as a place for teams to meet, administrative staff support, and time to fulfill the basic functions of the team, including regular meetings to exchange information and plan comprehensive interventions. Institutions

Table 28. Characteristics of Effective Interdisciplinary Teams

Institutional support

Shared philosophy, goals, and norms; goal directed

Effective leaders and leadership styles with emphasis on coordination

Emphasis on team interdependency with role recognition and support

Skilled communication and problem solving, especially when difficulties arise

Shared decision making

Flexibility and openness to new ideas

Documentation of care that ensures accountability and confidentiality

Effective collaboration with other healthcare providers, teams, and organizations

Formal team self-evaluation to improve future performance, ability to give effective feedback

Openness to discussing challenges, debriefing about difficult situations

Synergy, camaraderie, empowerment, and fun

should also recognize that regularly scheduled team evaluations and self-assessments to determine the team's effectiveness in terms of task and function are necessary. Evaluations and self-assessments should address the roles of the administrative staff, the management team, the IDT as a whole, and individual team members. Finally, recognition for achievements is an important aspect of institutional support, and the hospice and palliative care team can drive that recognition by creating and monitoring benchmarks for high-quality care.

The primary goal of hospice and palliative care teams is to alleviate the patient's and family's suffering, not to maintain the team. Adequate administrative support should be provided to establish and maintain a qualified, well-trained IDT of healthcare professionals to provide needed care. Executives, physicians, and managers may intentionally minimize the amount of time that they spend together, but members of teams need to be given enough time to learn to work together.[315]

Shared Principles, Goals, and Objectives

Depending on their size and maturity, hospice and palliative care programs are likely to use at least two types of teams: a management team and one or more interdisciplinary care teams. Effective IDTs agree on the team's guiding principles, its primary purpose and objectives, and expectations for each member.

Members of effective teams spend significant time and effort defining principles, purposes, and goals to which they subscribe both collectively and individually.[315] The principles, purposes, and many goals of hospice and palliative care IDTs are predetermined by the nature of the work. For example, members of IDTs must be committed to symptom control, relief of suffering, a team approach to whole-person care, and good communication. IDT members may have other goals, including educating medical students or serving specific populations, such as children or patients with HIV/AIDS.

Effective teams translate their purpose and goals into realistic, specific, measurable outcomes to evaluate their effectiveness. Examples of measurable outcome objectives include[332]

- reducing physical pain and other symptoms to acceptable levels within a specific number of hours or days
- measuring various events (eg, time to enrollment, arrival of medication, response to emergency calls, time to a death call)
- measuring patient and family satisfaction
- completing a healthcare power of attorney and living will documents at a certain rate
- documenting the number of IDT meetings that start on time, their attendance rates, and team satisfaction with these meetings.

Specific, measurable outcome objectives are powerful contributors to performance, job satisfaction, and an enhanced sense of purpose and meaning. Specific goals support clear communication, task-oriented conflict, and goal-directed care and are more likely to result in effective interventions. Measurable goals also provide tools to determine the effectiveness of a team's individual and collective interventions.[333]

Norms
All teams have norms, or unwritten rules that govern a group's behavior (ie, determining which behaviors are acceptable or unacceptable).[329,334] For example, people often sit in the same place at team meetings, and they will follow the norm and not sit in "the doctor's seat." Norms establish expectations for which course of action to take in certain situations.[322] For example, in a hospice team the first priority is patient comfort. This norm is well known by all team members and provides clear direction in the event of a pain crisis so that precious time is not lost while team members determine the best course of action.

If norms are allowed to form naturally, they can be destructive. Because group norms influence every aspect of how a team functions, it is best to intentionally structure an open discussion at the outset to clarify expectations and improve team functioning. It also can help to answer certain questions with your team such as the following:

- Is tardiness to meetings acceptable?
- Is doing paperwork during the meeting allowed?
- Are there assigned seats at IDT meetings?
- Is the meeting conversation dominated by one discipline?
- How should conflict between team members be handled?
- Is discussion of certain subjects prohibited?
- Are team members allowed to express their own feelings?
- Do all team members or only a few actively participate in team meetings?

- What does nonparticipation indicate in terms of honoring the specialized knowledge and expertise of each team member?
- Are IDT members allowed to set limits on their involvement to achieve a balanced life, or must they put patient care ahead of all other priorities, including interaction with their own families?

Effective Team Leadership and Leadership Styles

In an ideal situation, a team is a collective mind. It is a group of intelligent, devoted members with a common, clear, and elevating goal who collaborate to affect a positive outcome in their work. Assignment of a leader—or an individual directing the efforts of the group—at first appears to contradict the notion of a team. Yet without leadership most teams lack the necessary direction to attain their goal. This has been called the *team paradox*; leaders often are necessary to ensure teamwork, but their very existence threatens the team.[322] In routine healthcare settings, physicians often serve as leaders of IDTs. However, in the hospice and palliative care IDT setting, physicians routinely participate as colleagues. Leadership is often shared depending on the needs of specific situation.[324] Nevertheless, the patient's attending physician is medically and legally responsible for the patient's medical care, and the hospice medical director is ultimately responsible for the medical care of all patients.

In hospice and palliative care settings, the terms *leader* and *coordinator* are administrative labels that do not necessarily imply higher status or the right to make unilateral decisions.[252] For example, in many mature programs, the designated team meeting leader is likely to be a healthcare professional with strong organizational and facilitation skills and is not necessarily a physician. Regardless of who is appointed, effective team leaders exhibit the skills listed in **Table 29**.[327,329]

Table 29. Skills of Effective Leaders

Plan and facilitate meetings with clear objectives; meetings stay on track.

Encourage use of a problem-solving approach.

Ensure effective coordination and communication.

Share team decisions with necessary parties.

Keep extraneous anecdotal information to a minimum.

Help motivate team members to the highest possible standards of care.

Adapt leadership style to specific circumstances.

Balance problem-solving and task-oriented behavior with nurturing and motivating behavior.

Encourage regularly scheduled self-evaluations to measure the team's effectiveness in terms of its internal functioning and ability to alleviate suffering.

Effective IDTs may share leadership. For example, physicians are expected to provide leadership when the team is developing the medical component of a patient's care plan, but the social worker is expected to lead the development of a psychosocial care plan.

Effective leaders can adapt their leadership style to the needs of a specific group or situation. For example, a more autocratic, directive style might be appropriate for teams new to hospice and palliative care, but a democratic style is likely to be more effective for teams of seasoned hospice and palliative care professionals. Common leadership styles, each of which can be effective in specific situations, include the following:

- *Autocratic* leaders allow group members to have input but make the final decision.
- *Oligarchic* leaders appoint a small, specialized group to make final decisions.
- *Democratic* leaders ask group members to participate equally in decision making.
- *Laissez-faire* leaders allow group members to make their own decisions.

Team Interdependency with Role Recognition and Support

A high level of interdependence consistently enhances team performance.[335] Members of effective teams recognize that their ability to alleviate a patient's or family's suffering depends on the collective ability of the team. However, they also recognize the importance of individual responsibility and accountability. Effective teams

- recognize, honor, and use the expertise of each member of the team
- evaluate how each discipline can contribute to the team's overall goals
- recognize the need for role definition and role flexibility
- expect team members to represent their discipline's current practice standards and to participate fully in team meetings
- expect accountability for developing interventions and implementing interventions
- understand that a team's success depends on each member's ability to communicate effectively, work both independently and interdependently, and recognize individual and collective responsibilities
- provide support and ongoing training to maximize the team's effectiveness and the professional growth of each team member.

Team members should be familiar with the roles of other team members. For example, chaplains are not expected to be experts on assessing and managing pain, but they should be able to recognize signs of pain that is not being controlled and report the symptoms to the appropriate team member. Similarly, physicians are not expected to develop expertise in the assessment and treatment of spiritual pain, but they should be able to complete a preliminary assessment of spiritual pain as part of an overall history and discuss basic spiritual questions.

Role flexibility is essential when caring for dying patients and their families. Nurses and home healthcare aides often provide basic, supportive counseling for distressed patients and family members during home visits. Social workers and chaplains may need to help patients to the bathroom, straighten their sheets, or help them find more comfortable positions.

Role-related difficulties that affect performance and contribute to stress include role ambiguity, role conflict, and role overload.[329,334]

Role Ambiguity. Role ambiguity occurs when healthcare professionals are uncertain about how to participate in IDTs, when little or no orientation is provided, and when team members are expected to perform roles for which they have little or no education or training. Teams can reduce role ambiguity by discussing the roles of team members, listing all tasks associated with each role, and outlining areas of role uniqueness and overlap.[281,324] Role ambiguity is most likely to occur when

- traditional roles are adapted to nontraditional settings[329]
- roles and expectations are poorly defined or not clearly communicated
- priorities are not clearly communicated
- tasks are not clearly defined.

Role Conflict. Various types of conflict can occur among team members. However, conflict has both positive and negative influences on a team's productivity level. High-performing teams take advantage of "good" conflict, such as a principled debate about facts, challenging assertions, or playing devil's advocate. "Bad" conflict such as angry words, denial, lying, and gossip can be a threat to productivity.

According to Jehn, there are three types of conflict: relationship conflict involves disagreements based on personal and social issues not related to work; task conflict involves disagreements about work done in the group; and process conflict is disagreement regarding task strategy, delegation, and utilization of resources.[336] Typically task and process conflict improve team performance, but relationship conflict is destructive and can lead to increased burnout.[336,337]

Differing professional perspectives enhance the team's ability to provide comprehensive interventions. They also inevitably lead to conflicts about which interventions offer the best approach. When interrole conflicts are handled effectively, differences of opinion often result in interventions that better meet the patient and family's physical, social, emotional, and spiritual needs. Differences of opinion also provide team members with a better understanding of each discipline's perspective. However, unresolved, ongoing differences can lead to relationship conflict. This is more likely to occur when team members believe their contributions are consistently overlooked or team members believe their specific discipline serves a special patient advocacy role not shared by other disciplines.

Problem-based—not personality-based—discussions of patient-family problems can reduce the number of role conflicts.

Team members are likely to experience conflict. For example, the program's medical director is expected to provide expert symptom management and report to executive directors, boards, and, in the case of for-profit programs, owners and investors, all of whom are concerned with the program's financial health. When programs are reluctant to cover costs of the expensive palliative treatments sometimes needed to control difficult symptoms, the medical director may experience intrarole conflict. A physician may want to provide the most effective intervention regardless of cost, but the medical administrator may want to protect the program's financial health. On occasion, a medical director may insist on necessary but costly treatments or low patient-staff ratios, resulting in strained relationships with the program's administrators, owners, and investors.

Role Overload. Role overload most often occurs when team members are expected to complete an unrealistic amount of work in a given time frame or take on more responsibility without additional training or support. Team members can also bring role overload upon themselves by having unrealistic expectations of their own productivity levels.

Communication and Problem-Solving Skills
Teams depend on professional expertise, communication, and problem-solving skills to achieve their goals. Clear communication is essential; it provides the foundation on which the team's ability to function rests. Effective communication[113,338]

- enhances coordination
- facilitates the exchange of needed information
- advances the team's goals
- helps break down barriers
- improves understanding
- confirms and supports team members
- encourages ethical analysis
- respects everyone in the group
- helps listeners keep an open mind
- avoids profanity, sexism, and stereotypes.

Members of effective teams feel free to speak candidly and participate fully in team discussions. They also allow others to speak, respect the opinions of other team members, recognize the importance of thoroughly discussing each patient's situation (within reasonable time frames), and examine the burdens and benefits of suggested interventions.[339]

Ask for Clarification!

If there is ever any confusion about someone's role on the IDT, remember to always ask for clarification. This can help make sure everyone is on the same page regarding goals and expectations. For example, you could say, "Just so I know that we are on the same page, could you help me better understand your role when a patient is being discharged home with hospice?"

Clinical Situation

Ming

You are the hospice medical director attending the weekly hospice IDT meeting. Ming is a 48-year-old woman with metastatic breast cancer with bone metastases and severe pain. Mary, Ming's primary nurse, reports that her pain has been poorly controlled during the past week despite aggressive increases in morphine. Her dose is now double what it was only a week ago, and she is still crying out and looks miserable. She was seen by both a social worker and a chaplain this week, who both called the nurse to report her pain was uncontrolled. The nurse is asking you for assistance in addressing Ming's pain.

- Is there a process you can use to identify and resolve this issue with the IDT?
- How can you thoughtfully balance information gathered from all team members?

Team Decision Making

Making decisions regarding the care of patients is the primary function of the IDT. Despite the purest of intentions, teams of people will make poor decisions on a routine basis. It is critical to create a system within the team that allows for discussion and ongoing evaluation of decisions to enable the group to improve its performance over time and avoid repeating mistakes. Teams may follow a series of steps to help facilitate good decision making. These steps include

- defining the problem to be solved (addressing a pain crisis)
- setting the desired goals (goals should be measurable and have a clear time frame, such as a 50% reduction in a patient's pain within 48 hours)
- planning the group's process for decision making.

Ideal teams will then seek facts and reserve passing judgment until all the information is collected (eg, the IDT will hear from the nurse, social worker, chaplain, and bath aid without interruption, and the team leader takes notes on a whiteboard). After all the available and relevant information has been discussed, the team brainstorms possible interventions (eg, admitting the patient to an inpatient unit for subcutaneous or intravenous pain control, increasing oral opioids, adding adjuvant pain relievers, calling a family meeting with the patient's pastor, consulting with an anesthesiologist). After the options have been listed, the team discusses the merits of each and allows for open discussion. Finally the team makes a decision and recommends a course of action (eg, the nurse will admit the patient to the inpatient unit and will request a family meeting with the chaplain). In the near future, the group should revisit their decision and their decision-making process to evaluate their performance. Did the pain improve? Could their decision making have been better, given emergent information? The team should actively seek feedback from team members regarding the process and conduct a critical self-appraisal of their effectiveness.

The process of group decision making is generally a more time-consuming and involved process than that of an individual making a decision. Team decision making has the potential to consider a wide range of perspectives, which may improve the effectiveness of decisions and the consistency of group decisions. Because team decisions are more involved and take longer, teams can be advised to recognize situations that are best handled on an individual basis rather than as part of the team process. Teams can openly identify situations that should trigger a "team decision-making" process while recognizing that every decision an IDT makes is not necessarily a team decision. Forsyth proposed a model for rational group decision making that can help teams maintain focus and discipline through the process (**Figure 3**).[340]

Figure 3. A Model for the Team Decision-Making Process

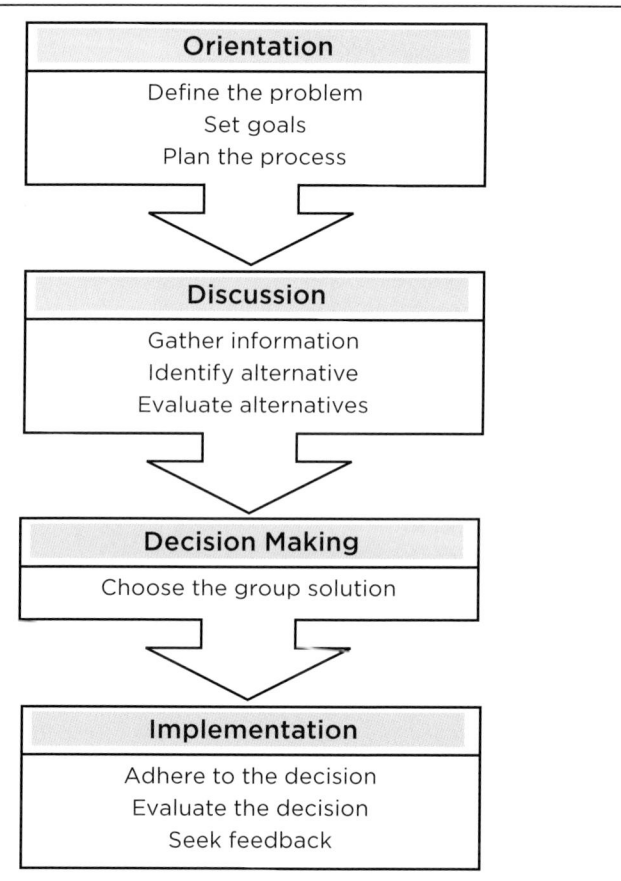

Orientation
Define the problem
Set goals
Plan the process

↓

Discussion
Gather information
Identify alternative
Evaluate alternatives

↓

Decision Making
Choose the group solution

↓

Implementation
Adhere to the decision
Evaluate the decision
Seek feedback

Republished with permission of Cengage Learning, from Group Dynamics, 2nd ed., by Forsyth DR, 2nd ed., 1990; permission conveyed through Copyright Clearance Center, Inc.

Shared Decision Making

IDTs rely on shared decision making. However, rapid changes in a patient's condition and acute needs of the patient or family may require immediate decisions by one or two members of the team. Emergency decisions are discussed later with the entire team. When groups of people make decisions, they generally use one or more of the methods listed in **Table 30**.

Openness to New Ideas

Members of effective teams understand that continuing education and openness to new ideas and perspectives are essential components of effective team performance and professional competence. Highly trained hospice and palliative care IDTs are subject to errors in judgment because of the "common knowledge effect." This is an observed phenomenon in which groups tend to discuss information they share rather than unique information.[341,342] There are some techniques that are useful—and some that are not—to minimize group susceptibility to the common information effect.[322] Ineffective strategies include

- increasing the amount of discussion
- separating the review phase from the discussion phase
- increasing the size of the group
- increasing the information load
- polling before the discussion.

Effective strategies include

- searching for and considering unique information
- defining the goal as a "problem to be solved," not a "judgment to be made"
- suspending initial judgment until after discussion
- having members write down facts during discussions that justify their decision

Table 30. Decision-Making Methods

Default. No decision is made (which is a decision). No one cares enough to voice an opinion, or team members are reluctant to voice an opinion because it is not politically expedient or it conflicts with spoken or unspoken group norms.

Unilateral. The most powerful person on the team (sometimes the team leader) makes the final decision.

Oligarchic. Decisions are made by a small group that may reverse or alter decisions made during the team meeting.

Majority rule. Members of the team vote and the majority wins, even if the decision is not in the best interests of the patient, family, or program. Before voting, team members should decide on the majority percentage (eg, 51% or 75%).

Unanimity. All members agree (or appear to agree) with a certain line of action.

Consensus. Discussion continues until all members reach a compromise even though no one may be completely satisfied with the final decision.

- ranking the options rather than choosing one
- considering alternatives independently
- minimizing status differences.

Formal Team Self-Evaluation
Like any other group or system, hospice and palliative care teams eventually develop lives of their own and begin to protect their own existence. To ensure the team's continued focus on alleviating patient and family distress, effective teams schedule regular self-assessments that focus on realistic goal attainment and team functioning. The team may choose to review its measurement goals to gain objective information on performance. It can also examine questions such as the following:
- Are the team's expectations realistic?
- Do interventions effectively alleviate the patient's and family's physical, spiritual, emotional, and social pain?
- How does the team measure its effectiveness?
- Are outcome measures used to determine progress toward specific goals?
- Is the team operating in the most efficient manner?
- Are all disciplines represented and accountable?
- Are roles as clearly defined as possible?
- Is the team developing dysfunctional behavioral patterns such as avoiding conflict at all costs, becoming professionally isolated, or spending more time on team maintenance rather than patient and family care?

Group process evaluation forms are available. One form that can be used to evaluate team function is the Sample Group Process Assessment Form from Carnegie Mellon University (https://www.cmu.edu/teaching/designteach/teach/instructionalstrategies/groupprojects/tools/index.html; Accessed April 27, 2017).

If challenges in communication with team members arise, it may be helpful to utilize the DiSC personal assessment tool to evaluate individual communication styles. For example, a type D (Dominance) personality tends to make quick decisions and seek immediate results, while a type I (Influence) likes to collaborate and dislikes being ignored. Tailoring communication to a colleague's particular style may improve collaboration and reduce conflict.[343]

Synergy, Camaraderie, Empowerment, and Fun
There are certain stresses that inevitably result when caring for terminally ill patients. Effective teams combat these stresses with good morale, support, and encouragement. Members of effective teams support each other and temporarily lighten each other's load when personal difficulties or work-related stresses arise, and there is evidence to support the use of team huddles to clarify roles and offload burden.[344] Effective teams realize that no one member is indispensable; this allows members to leave at the end of the day confident that others will care for patients during their absence. Effective teams also recognize the importance of

positive feedback and recognition to promote team performance, as well as the importance of professional and personal growth and appropriate humor (see Use Appropriate Humor on page 26).[330]

Threats to Team Performance

Table 31 describes common problems and barriers to effective teamwork.[330,339]

Table 31. Common Problems and Barriers to Effective Teamwork

Breakdown in Eliciting Information

Teams need to gather enough information to make good decisions about treatment. When team leaders use only closed questions or brief assertions, it is unlikely that other team members will provide enough information to make good decisions; for example, "Did you order that?" "Do you want the patient to think we don't care?"

Promotional Leadership

Promotional leadership occurs when team leaders or powerful team members voice an idea or opinion before asking for team input; this affects the candor of the team and usually occurs unintentionally, but it can be used in a subtle way to prevent or limit discussion while appearing to be open minded. An example, "I think we should transfer this patient back home immediately. Now I'd like to hear what you think."

Private Agendas

Periodic conflict is expected because effective teams are candid and often debate the best interventions to use in specific situations. Effective team members "tell it like it is" and sometimes argue. They are not always cautious, nor do they make safe, innocuous comments or suggestions. However, when private agendas develop and cliques occur, candor disappears, asking for information becomes a method to demean team members, and one-upmanship replaces teamwork.

Insufficient Alternatives

Failure to explore all options before making decisions can prematurely close discussion and result in the team's wishing it had spent more time discussing alternatives before taking action. Although exploring alternatives is time consuming, it generally results in better ideas and decisions.

Lack of Candor

Good decisions are based on complete information, which requires accurate disclosure of relevant information by all team members. Barriers to candor include personal reasons for not being honest (not wanting to hurt someone's feelings or put someone on the spot) and team politics (team members may distort information because it is the expedient thing to do). Challenges to the team's values, norms, goals, and objectives should be honored.

Continued on page 112

Table 31. Common Problems and Barriers to Effective Teamwork (continued)

Lack of Ongoing Self-Assessment
Lack of careful analysis of the team's functioning and effectiveness can lead to scapegoating—for example, an unpopular person is viewed as causing all the team's problems. Regularly scheduled self-assessments should address the team's strengths, weaknesses, and functioning.

Lack of Responsibility
The emphasis on collective team responsibility and shared leadership can result in lack of individual accountability and ineffective leadership. Overdependence on team members leads to a loss of personal responsibility, accountability, and independence.

Unresolved Conflict
Ongoing disagreements about policies often generate conflict; for example, assigned tasks cannot be completed within usual working hours. When constant self-sacrifice is required, the program's structure and staffing should be examined. Good patient care should not depend on team members' ongoing willingness to devalue other aspects of their lives, such as marital and family relationships, spiritual and religious growth, and self-care activities.

Failure to Communicate Team Decisions to Others
Even when excellent plans are generated, they are unlikely to succeed unless all parties are willing to collaborate. Team decisions must be effectively communicated to those who implement plans, such as home health aides, volunteers, and home care nurses.

Name the Conflict

As with any emotional situation, using empathetic communications skills is helpful in managing team conflicts. One tool is to simply name the conflict. For example, you could say, "It seems that we're not agreeing on the appropriate next step here. At the same time, it's clear we're both trying to honor the patient's wishes. I can see how stressful this disagreement has been. I really value your insight into this situation. Perhaps we could sit together and think about a solution that will meet the patient's needs and make sense to both of us?"

Signs and Symptoms of Dysfunctional Teams

All groups operate in ways that support or impede the group's goals. Even functional groups often become temporarily dysfunctional when stressors occur, such as changes in membership, changes in funding, and dysfunctional behavior of an important group member. Symptoms of dysfunctional team behavior may be difficult to assess because of denial or reluctance to admit the team is becoming dysfunctional, helplessness or uncertainty about how to intervene, or lack of awareness of the symptoms of dysfunctional team behavior. The sooner the symptoms of dysfunctional team behavior are recognized and interventions are implemented, the more likely the team will be to return to healthy functioning. **Table 32** describes selected symptoms of dysfunctional teams.[345,346]

Table 32. Symptoms of Dysfunctional Teams

Closed vs Open Structure

Closed structure is likely when team members think of themselves as "us" and everyone else as "them." Members of closed teams are fearful of people who want to attend team meetings if those people are not viewed as members of the "official" team, such as a patient's family member, minister, or nursing home or hospital staff person who cares for the patient.

The Team Leader Becomes Dysfunctional

In the long run, "one-person" IDTs that rely on the skills of a charismatic team member are ineffective. The following behaviors are characteristic of dysfunctional leadership behavior:
- The leader does not allow questions about decisions.
- The leader takes credit for all the program's success and blames others for its failures.
- The leader schedules team meetings at times that exclude certain members, such as attending physicians.
- The leader forms inappropriate relationships with certain team members.

Team or Program Isolation from the Rest of the Healthcare Community

Collaboration with other healthcare providers is limited or nonexistent, team members are suspicious of other healthcare providers, access to outside professional organizations is limited, or professional travel is restricted to a few favored members of the team. Team members socialize exclusively with one another and believe that only they understand the stresses of working with dying patients. Team members believe the special nature of working with patients with terminal illness absolves them from professional ethical guidelines and/or emotional presence in other relationships (eg, marital or parental roles).

Self-Perpetuation and Homogenization of Members or Staff

Team members are recruited only from within the team's social network.

Isolation and Scapegoating of Unpopular Team Members

Team members who question policies, decisions, or group norms are isolated.

All Problems Projected onto a Common Outside Enemy

Blame for all the team's problems is projected onto funding sources, other healthcare organizations, computer systems, unpopular managers, or members of the community.

Increased Interpersonal Conflict

Unresolved conflicts lead to passive-aggressive behavior instead of conflict resolution, gossip instead of direct communication, and increased turnover as members who are unwilling to work in a dysfunctional setting leave for other positions.

Absenteeism

Frequent absences indicate that team meetings are no longer meeting the needs of team members.

Continued on page 114

Table 32. Symptoms of Dysfunctional Teams (continued)

Outsourcing of Care
Frequent outsourcing of care and overuse of inpatient care can be a sign of inadequate training or lack of time to provide effective care (eg, all anxious or depressed patients are immediately referred to a psychiatrist).

Focus Shifts from Patient Care to the Team's Personal and Interpersonal Problems
As team dysfunction increases, meetings consume much of the work week and energy is directed to resolving conflicts, providing team support, and maintaining the team. Patient care is not adequately addressed because the team's energy is being expended on its own problems.

Development of Problematic Social and Sexual Relationships Between Team Members or Team Members and Patients
Inappropriate social and sexual relationships are indicators of serious dysfunction.

Managing Team Conflict

There are several approaches to managing interpersonal team conflict.[290,347]

- During the discussion, it is important for both parties to respect the other person and work together to develop possible solutions.
- As soon as emotions have cooled, deal with the problem instead of waiting.
- Meet in a private area that will be free from interruptions.
- Describe what happened; for example, "I was not told that my patient, Mrs. Smith, died over the weekend."
- Describe the emotional consequences; for example, "On Monday morning I was embarrassed when I went to Mrs. Smith's house for a home visit. Her husband told me she was dead and said I should know more about my patients."
- Specify what you want to happen in the future and how you can help; for example, "I think home healthcare nurses should be better informed about weekend events."
- Describe the consequences if behavior is changed; for example, "There will be better communication and less confusion on Monday mornings."
- Work together to generate possible solutions; for example, "We could work with a small group of involved parties and draft a procedure for communicating weekend events."
- Choose an agreed-upon solution.
- Form a plan, try it for a period of time, and evaluate its effectiveness.

Skills to Facilitate Conflict Resolution

When conflicts cannot be resolved by involved parties, outside intervention may be required. In these cases, third-party facilitators should use conflict-resolution skills that include the following:

- Welcome the existence of conflict, bring it into the open, and use it as the basis for positive change.
- Clarify the nature of the problem. Is this the real problem?

- Reduce the areas of conflict. List specific problems and confine the discussion to problems identified by both parties.
- Suggest procedures and ground rules.
- Identify short- and long-term goals.
- Identify factors that keep the individuals in conflict.
- Suggest and then evaluate as many solutions as possible, looking for those that preserve each party's dignity and self-esteem.
- Agree on one solution, record it, and ensure that both parties agree on the meaning of the solution as it is written.
- Try the solution and then reevaluate it.

Giving Feedback

Although learners and faculty often acknowledge that giving and receiving feedback is important, many often feel poorly prepared to provide feedback.[348] When working as part of an IDT, a key element of effective communication and team functioning is the ability to give targeted, nonjudgmental feedback. Giving feedback can help clarify expectations and improve performance while encouraging a culture of support and excellence.[349] Ideally any member of the IDT should feel comfortable giving feedback to any other member.

Feedback should be given immediately, and it should be clear that time is being taken to provide feedback.[350,351] Saying something such as "Would it be okay if I gave you some feedback on what I noticed?" may be a helpful transition. Comments should focus on specific observations instead of general statements. For example, "I really liked how you said 'a prognosis of weeks to months'" instead of "I liked how you gave the prognosis." Start by mentioning a positive observation and then transition into one or two specific ways for improvement. As with any discussion of serious news, sometimes receiving feedback may be considered "bad news." As such, expect emotional reactions when giving feedback and respond with empathy. Sometimes asking for bidirectional feedback can be helpful.[352] **Table 33** illustrates some qualities of effective feedback.

Giving feedback to a colleague is often a sensitive issue. It can be seen as critical or judgmental and may not be perceived with the intended effect of improving skills and enhancing patient care. Acknowledging the awkwardness of providing feedback in this situation is helpful (naming the emotion), and focusing feedback on the specific observations and not the individual is recommended. The following is an example of giving feedback to a colleague in an IDT setting.

> **RN:** *Thank you for being here for the family meeting, I think it was very helpful. Would it be okay if I gave you some feedback based on my experience with the family?*
>
> **MD:** *Yes, please.*
>
> **RN:** *I think the way you used clear, nonmedical terms in your discussion was very effective for the family. They almost always have questions after the doctor leaves, I think they are a little too overwhelmed to ask during the meetings. I felt like there were times when they seemed to have questions today. Maybe pausing every so often and seeing if there are any questions might be helpful for them next time? What do you think?*

Table 33. Qualities of Effective Feedback

Clear transition to giving feedback

Ask for permission to give feedback

Timely, immediately after

Specific, focused on observed behaviors instead of personality traits

Honest

Nonjudgmental

Balanced, including both positive and corrective elements

Linked to learner's goals (if providing feedback to learner)

Avoids the "feedback sandwich," which can give mixed messages

Interactive (ask learner to assess his/her performance first)

Coping with Stress

Difficult Encounters

Difficult encounters with patients and family members raise powerful emotions in care providers and present their own set of major challenges. When physicians must care for these types of patients, it is important to acknowledge several factors. First, not all patients with terminal illness are calm and friendly; some are abusive and manipulative. Remember that we usually are not the cause of a patient's or family member's anger. Physicians are likely to experience some degree of dislike, anger, and revulsion when confronted with manipulative behaviors from patients or family members who refuse to implement agreed-upon interventions. Physicians are likely to avoid patients and family members they do not like and later feel guilty about not establishing a therapeutic relationship. Consequently it is not only difficult to establish therapeutic relationships with patients and family members displaying anger or abusive behaviors, but it is also difficult to establish and maintain a minimal professional relationship.[353,354]

Physicians can try several strategies when working in these difficult situations. They can make a conscious effort to find some common ground with the patient. They can use open-ended questions and allow patients to talk more, helping to elicit their life story and shed light on their behavior.[355] Sometimes an angry patient simply needs a nonjudgmental outlet for his anger. In this situation, active listening and responding with empathy while the patient vents may be helpful. Physicians can also use self-knowledge, self-monitoring, and self-evaluation to better understand personal issues that may be contributing to strong emotional reactions to certain patients.[355]

When it becomes clear that a satisfying patient-physician relationship is not going to occur regardless of the physician's best efforts, several strategies can be implemented. For example, try to establish some emotional distance from the patient. Concentrate on acting in a professional manner. Taking time for self-care activities will help reduce stress and maintain some sense of perspective. Try involving other team members, some of whom might be able to develop more effective relationships with specific patients. If necessary, refer the patient to another physician.[355]

Burnout

Most hospice and palliative medicine physicians view themselves as healers (more so than identifying as technicians, purveyors of pills, or "proceduralists") and are troubled when they cannot establish satisfying relationships with patients and family members. When too many stressors occur simultaneously, however, stress overload compromises a physician's judgment and interferes with the ability to interact compassionately with patients, families, and coworkers.[356,357] **Table 34** lists organizational, professional, and personal stressors frequently associated with stress overload. **Table 35**[358] describes signs and symptoms of stress overload in physicians.

> **"I'm going to sue you!"**
> Sometimes emotions become so heated that family members threaten to seek legal representation. Perhaps this reaction is from legitimate concerns of inappropriate medical care or from any number of complicated emotions. Regardless, supporting the family with empathy is advised. It is also advised to make risk management and hospital legal counsel aware of the situation. Acknowledgment of blame is not necessary.
>
> Consider saying the following: "I can't imagine what you are going through right now. I can sense how upset and disappointed you are with the medical care, and that you love your father dearly. You are being an amazing advocate for your father."
>
> The strategic use of silence (letting the person vent his anger) is another useful approach.

Stress-Management Strategies

Frederic Hudson, a psychologist working in the field of adult renewal, has identified a set of core values with which we can organize our lives and sustain and renew ourselves.[360] He characterizes these core values as having to do with a sense of self:

- intimacy
- achievement
- creativity and play
- search for meaning
- compassion and contribution.

To provide a strong sense of self, one must take care of body and mind. Taking care of oneself—whether through exercise, vacation, meditation, or pleasure reading—is a standard we all must work to attain. Intimacy refers to the invigorating power of personal relationships with our family members, friends, and colleagues that can recharge our worn spirit. External recognition for our work is only part of the sense of achievement Hudson refers to; an internal directive to improve the world around us through good works can provide a more meaningful sense of achievement. Do not neglect the need for nonworking vacations, good art of any kind, or the redemptive and regenerative power of sitting in a quiet room and journaling or writing prose or poetry.[361]

As a start, consider your most important values for a moment. Physicians help patients explore their own life story and goals; why not search for meaning in our own existence to renew our passion for caring for the dying? Compassion for our fellow human beings is a shared trait for many end-of-life practitioners. Rewarding those around us contributes positive energy to the group, provides recognition, and helps justify our collective efforts.[362]

Table 34. Factors Associated with Stress Overload Among Physicians[358]

Personal Variables

Age. Young age is associated with more stress, fewer coping mechanisms, and more burnout.

Personality. People with hardy personalities often cope better with work-related stress. They view change as a normal challenge that contributes to further development. Hardy personalities are characterized by commitment, challenge, curiosity about life and meaning, and a sense of being able to influence events.

Motivation for career choice. Paradoxically, the reasons for choosing palliative medicine can contribute to stress overload. For example, a desire to help others contributes to stress when the physician's help is not wanted or appreciated. In some cases, physicians devote so much energy to their patients that they have none left for themselves or their family members.[359]

Social supports. Physicians who use only their own family members for emotional support and debriefing are likely to experience difficulties when family members are unable or unwilling to continue providing sole support (eg, when family members experience their own crises).

Life events. Stressful life events (for example, family illness, bereavement, or relationship problems create additional stress and can contribute to stress overload.)

Role Difficulties

Role ambiguity, excessive responsibility, and role conflict create stress.

Communication Problems

Communication problems with peers, team members, patients, the patient's family members, and the physician's family members contribute to stress.

Difficulty expressing deep pain and grief when interventions fail to relieve a patient's suffering or when favorite patients die can lead to unexpressed, unacknowledged grief that accumulates over time.

Organizational Stresses

Inadequate resources and staffing, professional isolation and the loneliness associated with practicing in a developing field of medicine, and conflicts with program managers and/or owners all may contribute to stress for physicians.

Perhaps most critical of all for renewal is our own mindset, suggested by Hatem to be the most powerful means of motivation.[363] Viktor Frankl, the Viennese psychiatrist, writes about choosing to stay with his Austrian family in the dark days of World War II despite having a visa that would have allowed him entry into the United States. The concentration camps followed; in surviving them, his assertion becomes all the more poignant. "Anything can be taken from a man," he wrote, "but one thing: the last of human freedoms—to choose one's attitude in any given set of circumstances, to choose one's own way."[364]

When caring for terminally ill patients, physicians must learn to acknowledge their own needs and anticipate the inevitable occurrence of psychological and spiritual issues that will

Table 35. Signs and Symptoms of Stress Overload Among Physicians[358]

Tiredness out of proportion to the work that is being done

Low morale

Over conscientiousness, loss of a sense of proportion, and preoccupation with patients

Loss of sense of humor

Conflicts with staff and scapegoating

Avoidance of patients

Difficulties at home

Distancing, depersonalization, and intellectualization

Anger, irritability, and frustration

Helplessness, inadequacy, and insecurity

Depression, grief, and guilt

Errors in judgment

---

cause them personal distress.[365] When events threaten to overwhelm their resources for coping, physicians need to recognize the importance of the following: ministering to body, mind, and spirit; making specific plans for self-care; and acting on these plans.[366] Mindfulness techniques and deep breathing exercises may be helpful,[367,368] while strategies such as those described in **Table 36** can help reduce stress and enhance personal and professional growth. There are also strategies available for building resilience in the team through specific resiliency training programs that involve cognitive behavioral therapy and positive psychology techniques.[369]

With the help of self-care activities and spiritual practices such as nature appreciation, reflective reading and writing, contemplative prayer, meditation, and yoga, physicians can learn to transcend their own role attachments and coexist with the normal feelings of fear, guilt, and grief. Physicians who accept their own periodic bouts of psychological and spiritual distress are better able to empathize with the psychological pain experienced by patients with terminal illness as they try to come to terms with loss in new and more meaningful ways.

Self-care and self-awareness practices and resources that have been helpful to other palliative care physicians are presented in **Table 37**.

Dr. Cicely Saunders reminds physicians that dying patients need the support of a caring community, and the community needs the insights of dying patients. As healthcare professionals witness the attempts of patients with terminal illness to develop a renewed sense of meaning, purpose, and hope, they are frequently inspired to examine their own sources of meaning. Few professional opportunities offer such great rewards.

Table 36. Strategies to Manage Stress[358]

Develop a Sense of Competence

Develop professional skills, set realistic goals, test competence in a number of different situations, and share competence with others.

Attend palliative medicine conferences.

Locate resources for assistance with difficult cases (eg, call AAHPM to receive help locating other hospice and palliative care physicians with similar interests).

Develop Practice Patterns that Enhance Control and Pleasure

Focus on areas of personal interest and schedule appointments so difficult patients are followed by enjoyable or fulfilling cases and patients.

Develop Decision-Making Protocols

Develop formal decision-making protocols, particularly when making difficult treatment-related decisions.

Involve others in the decision-making process (see *UNIPAC 6*).

Develop Collegial Relationships with Other Professionals

Develop supportive relationships with physicians and other healthcare professionals to alleviate isolation and provide sources of professional and emotional support.

Discuss painful psychological and spiritual issues with others (eg, interested peers, clergy, counselors).

Develop Staffing Policies that Reduce Stress

Establish policies that allow adequate time away from the work setting.

Develop a Personal Philosophy that Provides a Sense of Meaning[370]

Develop a personal philosophy that provides a sense of meaning for illness, death, and the physician's own role.

Develop Strategies that Provide a Sense of Rejuvenation

Participate in activities that provide a sense of psychological, physical, and spiritual rejuvenation (eg, meditation, prayer, worship, exercise, enjoying the outdoors).

Use religious and spiritual practices to strengthen the clinician's spiritual resources.

Spend time with family members, not only doing productive things but also just being together.

Participate in activities for their intrinsic enjoyment, not for reward or acclamation (eg, read nonprofessional literature, listen to or play music, garden, walk, watch birds, write poetry).

Develop Personal Habits that Increase the Ability to Cope with Stress

Get adequate sleep and frequent exercise and develop healthy eating patterns.

Balance work and home life to avoid exhaustion.[365]

Use counseling to gain insights and to help to resolve problems.

Get enough time off from being on-call and take vacations whenever possible.

Continued on page 122

Table 36. Strategies to Manage Stress[358] (continued)

Acknowledge Life's Imperfections

Acknowledge the likelihood of periodic challenges to the clinician's psychological and spiritual equilibrium.

Recognize limitations and the inability to ensure a perfect outcome for every patient and family.

Recognize that effectively using available knowledge and resources, providing caring presence, and referring to team members and consultants is all that can be done.

If Necessary, Find New Professional Opportunities

When coping mechanisms fail and external situations cannot be changed, it may be necessary to leave unhealthy work situations and find other, more satisfying professional opportunities.

Table 37. Suggested Self-Care and Self-Awareness Workplace Practices

Self-Care and Mindfulness Techniques[a]

As you walk from your car to your workplace or through the corridors of your workplace, attend carefully to the sensation of contact between your feet and the ground.

Set your watch or telephone alarm for midday each day. Use this as a prompt to perform some simple act of centering; for example, take four deep, slow breaths; think of a loved one; recite a favorite line of poetry or a prayer; or imagine weights around your waist and the words "ground, down."

Reward yourself after the completion of a task, for example, with an early coffee break.

Call a "time out" (usually just a few minutes) as a way of dealing with emotional flooding after a traumatic event; call a colleague to say, "I need a walk," or take a break. Stop at a window in your workplace and notice something in nature; consciously give it your full attention for a few moments.

Take half a minute of silence or take turns to choose and read a poem at the beginning of weekly IDT meetings. Before going into the next patient's room, pause and bring your attention to the sensation of your breathing for two to five breaths.

Take a snack before the end of clinic to prevent neuroglycopenia.

Stay connected to the outside world during the day; for example, check in with loved ones.

Multitask self-care; for example, dictate or meditate while using a treadmill in your office.

Continued on page 123

Table 37. Suggested Self-Care and Self-Awareness Workplace Practices (continued)

Use the suggested 20 seconds of hand washing in creative ways; for example, pay attention to the sensation of the water on your skin and allow yourself to sink into this experience; make this an act of conscious receiving by acknowledging to yourself, "I am worthy of my own time"; repeat a favorite line from a poem or prayer; or sing yourself "Happy Birthday!"

Don't be afraid to ask the question, "Is it time for a break?"

Deliberately make connections during the day with colleagues and with patients; for example, use humor, look for something particular or unusual in the patient's room, or notice patient's birth date or age.

Keep a notebook and write "field notes" on traumatic or meaningful encounters and events; occasionally take time at IDT meetings to share this material.

Write a "55-word story" in which you think about a topic or experience, and write freely for 5-10 minutes. Then spend another 5-10 minutes editing the passage down to exactly 55 words.

Deliberately develop a "role-shedding ritual" at the end of the day; for example, pay attention to putting away your stethoscope or hanging up your white coat.

Use the drive home from work deliberately; for example, take the longer, more interesting route; listen attentively to the news, music, or books on tape.

The following are verbatim descriptions of self-care practices from a sample of experienced clinicians, some of whom have been working in end-of-life care for more than 30 years:
- "I recite the words 'make me an instrument of thy peace' as I approach the hospital and before going into a situation I do not know how to handle."
- "I always try to figure out some way to touch the patient during the visit…shake hands, do even a small part of the physical exam. When I check the blood pressure, I hold the patient's arm in between my side and my arm, which is both an accurate and intimate technique that helps me feel really connected."
- "While taking blood pressure, I ask patients to breathe slowly through their nose, and I mirror their breathing with my own."
- "I practice daily meditation before leaving my office for rounds or clinic."
- "I pause mindfully prior to each new patient or new intervention, for example, while scrubbing prior to each surgical operation. I silently acknowledge my fellow-traveler connection to the patient prior to our discussion. I consciously monitor my sense of inner stress during the encounter and respond by intentionally returning to the place of quiet within, by briefly focusing on the lower retrosternal region. I visualize a healing connection (my wife, dog, friend) as I move between patients."
- "As I wash my hands I say to myself, 'May the universal life force enable me to treat my patients and colleagues with compassion, patience, and respect.'"

Continued on page 124

Table 37. Suggested Self-Care and Self-Awareness Workplace Practices (continued)

Web Resources[b]

Self-Awareness and Self-Care

Professional Quality of Life Scale	http://www.proqol.org/ProQol_Test.html	This is a short (30-item) self-test that physicians and other practitioners can use to gauge their level of compassion satisfaction, burnout, and compassion fatigue.
Commonweal	https://www.commonweal.org/	Education and training center that offers retreat workshops for physicians aimed at enhancing wellness and a sense of meaning in medicine.
Center for Practitioner Renewal	http://www.practitionerrenewal.ca/	Center for research on mental health and well-being in the healthcare workplace that offers consultation, counseling, supervision, and education programs for physicians.

Mindfulness Meditation

Spirit Rock Meditation Center	https://spiritrock.org/	Offers ongoing classes, day-long programs, and residential retreats about insight or mindfulness meditation.
University of Massachusetts Medical School Center for Mindfulness in Medicine, Health Care, and Society	www.umassmed.edu/cfm/mindfulness-based-programs/mbsr-courses/	Offers mindfulness meditation–based stress-reduction programs and education and research programs on mindfulness meditation.
The Institute for Poetic Medicine	www.poeticmedicine.org	The use of both reading and writing poetry as a therapeutic process in medicine.
Center for Civic Reflection	civicreflection.org	The use of reflective reading exercises to facilitate exploration of art and culture as it relates to the work of healthcare professionals, and to search for deeper meaning in and understanding of daily experiences.

[a]Based on the experiences of the authors and their colleagues, and various mindfulness techniques.
[b]Websites accessed April 27, 2017.
Reproduced with permission from JAMA. 2009. 301(11): 1155-1164. Copyright©2009 American Medical Association. All rights reserved.[371]

Summary

Engel argues that the most necessary and the most complex skills of the physician are the ability to elicit an accurate verbal account of the patient's illness experience and then to analyze it properly. He believes that it takes a careful discipline to develop reliable skills in the interviewing process and to understand "the meaning" of the patient's report in psychological, social, and cultural as well as anatomical, physiological, or biochemical terms.[122]

—Williamson and Noel

Stories are medicine.... They have such power; they do not require that we do, be, act anything—we need only listen. The remedies for repair or reclamation of any lost psychic drive are contained in stories. Stories engender the excitement, sadness, questions, longings, and understandings that spontaneously bring the archetype back to the surface....Stories set the inner life into motion, and this is particularly important where the inner life is frightened, wedged, or cornered. Story greases the hoists and pulleys, it causes adrenaline to surge, shows us the way out, down, or up, and for our trouble, cuts for us fine wide doors in previously blank walls, openings that lead to the dreamland, that lead to love and learning, that lead us back to our own real lives.[372]

—Clarissa Pinkola Estés

There is a growing recognition that communication skills are not only important but teachable.[137,373-375] Several educational programs centered around principles similar to those delineated in this book have been effective in improving healthcare provider attitudes and skills.[8,107-110,376-378] Effective training techniques to improve communication include those listed in **Table 38**; however, skills training alone may not be enough. Beneficial behavior changes are more likely to occur when skills training is coupled with exercises that enhance personal growth and awareness.[379] Multiple peer-reviewed curricula exist that can be used as teaching guides when educating learners. Some of these are included in **Table 39**.

Table 38. Training for Effective Communication

Read books and attend conferences on effective communication.[380]

Use interactive video recordings instead of audio tapes, because they more effectively illustrate nonverbal communication.

Attend small-group training sessions on effective communication.

Videotape interactions with simulated patients, and receive feedback from experienced facilitators.

Videotape interactions with terminally ill patients and receive feedback from experienced facilitators.

Table 39. Curricular Resources for Teaching Communication Skills[a]

Association of American Medical Colleges MedEdPORTAL	https://www.mededportal.org
• Breaking Bad News	https://www.mededportal.org/publication/10015[381]
• OSCE for communicating poor prognosis	https://www.mededportal.org/publication/9700[382]
• Breaking Bad News using RolePlay	https://www.mededportal.org/publication/9798[383]
The Stanford School of Medicine Palliative Care Training Portal	https://palliative.stanford.edu/
Vital Talk	www.vitaltalk.org/
	https://itunes.apple.com/us/app/vital-talk/id639969220?mt=8
	https://play.google.com/store/apps/details?id=org.vitaltalk.tips&hl=en

[b]Websites accessed April 27, 2017.

As patients, families, and physicians confront the unfathomable mysteries of life and death, hospice and palliative medicine requires
- excellent skills in palliative medicine
- an ability to communicate with honesty and compassion
- an ability to work with other healthcare professionals to alleviate the physical, emotional, spiritual, and social contributors to the suffering often experienced by terminally ill patients and their families
- an abiding interest in patients and their stories[384]
- an ability to let go of the need to always be in control
- a willingness to periodically let go of the role of teacher and become the student.

Alleviating a patient's physical, emotional, spiritual, and social pain in the context of a terminal illness requires excellent communication skills and an interdisciplinary approach to care. As dying patients struggle to find a renewed sense of meaning, purpose, value, self-worth, and hope for their lives, they want to understand their illness not only cognitively but also emotionally and spiritually. They want more than facts about their diagnosis, prognosis, and treatment plan. They want guidance, compassionate understanding, and a chance to tell their stories. In the midst of all the talking that goes on in their lives, patients long for understanding and the deep emotional and spiritual healing that accompanies true communication and the sense of being heard.[385]

References

1. Katz J. *The Silent World of Doctor and Patient*. Baltimore, MD: Johns Hopkins University Press; 2002.
2. Hampton JR, Harrison MJ, Mitchell JR, Prichard JS, Seymour C. Relative contributions of history-taking, physical examination, and laboratory investigation to diagnosis and management of medical outpatients. *Br Med J*. 1975;2(5969):486-489.
3. Peterson MC, Holbrook JH, Von Hales D, Smith NL, Staker LV. Contributions of the history, physical examination, and laboratory investigation in making medical diagnoses. *West J Med*. 1992;156(2):163-165.
4. Irwin WG, McClelland R, Love AH. Communication skills training for medical students: an integrated approach. *Med Educ*. 1989;23(4):387-394.
5. Epstein RM, Street R. L. J. Patient-Centered Communication in Cancer Care: Promoting Healing and Reducing Suffering. Bethesda, MD: National Cancer Institute, NIH Publication No. 07-6225; 2007. https://healthcaredelivery.cancer.gov/pcc/pcc_monograph.pdf?file=/pcc/communication/pcc_monograph.pdf. Accessed April 28, 2017.
6. Stagno SJ, Zhukovsky DS, Walsh D. Bioethics: communication and decision-making in advanced disease. *Semin Oncol*. 2000;27(1):94-100.
7. King A, Hoppe RB. "Best practice" for patient-centered communication: a narrative review. *J Grad Med Educ*. 2013;5(3):385-393.
8. Gustin J, Stowers KH, von Guten CF. Communication education for physicians. In: Wittenberg E, Ferrell BR, Goldsmith J, Smith T, Glajchen M, Handzo GF, eds. *Textbook of Palliative Care Communication* New York, NY: Oxford University Press; 2015:355.
9. Beach MC, Inui T. Relationship-centered care. A constructive reframing. *J Gen Intern Med*. 2006;21 Suppl 1:S3-8.
10. Institute of Medicine. Crossing the Quality Chasm: A New Health System for the 21st Century. Washington, DC: National Academy Press; 2001. https://www.nap.edu/read/10027/chapter/1. Accessed April 12, 2017.
11. Alston C, Paget L, Halvorson G, et al. Communicating with patients on health care evidence. IOM Roundtable on Value & Science-Driven Health Care; September, 2012; Washington, DC. https://nam.edu/wp-content/uploads/2015/06/VSRT-Evidence.pdf. Accessed April 28, 2017.
12. Temel JS, Greer JA, Muzikansky A, et al. Early palliative care for patients with metastatic non-small-cell lung cancer. *N Engl J Med*. 2010;363(8):733-742.
13. Dimoska A, Butow PN, Dent E, Arnold B, Brown RF, Tattersall MH. An examination of the initial cancer consultation of medical and radiation oncologists using the Cancode interaction analysis system. *Br J Cancer*. 2008;98(9):1508-1514.
14. Steinhauser KE, Alexander SC, Byock IR, George LK, Olsen MK, Tulsky JA. Do preparation and life completion discussions improve functioning and quality of life in seriously ill patients? Pilot randomized control trial. *J Palliat Med*. 2008;11(9):1234-1240.
15. Fawole OA, Dy SM, Wilson RF, et al. A systematic review of communication quality improvement interventions for patients with advanced and serious illness. *J Gen Intern Med*. 2013;28(4):570-577.
16. Bernacki RE, Block SD. Communication about serious illness care goals: a review and synthesis of best practices. *JAMA Intern Med*. 2014;174(12):1994-2003.
17. Zolnierek KB, Dimatteo MR. Physician communication and patient adherence to treatment: a meta-analysis. *Med Care*. 2009;47(8):826-834.
18. Lilly CM, De Meo DL, Sonna LA, et al. An intensive communication intervention for the critically ill. *Am J Med*. 2000;109(6):469-475.

19. Reader TW, Flin R, Cuthbertson BH. Communication skills and error in the intensive care unit. *Curr Opin Crit Care*. 2007;13(6):732-736.
20. Levinson W, Roter DL, Mullooly JP, Dull VT, Frankel RM. Physician-patient communication. The relationship with malpractice claims among primary care physicians and surgeons. *JAMA*. 1997;277(7):553-559.
21. Morrison RS, Penrod JD, Cassel JB, et al. Cost savings associated with US hospital palliative care consultation programs. *Arch Intern Med*. 2008;168(16):1783-1790.
22. Fujimori M, Shirai Y, Asai M, et al. Development and preliminary evaluation of communication skills training program for oncologists based on patient preferences for communicating bad news. *Palliat Support Care*. 2014;12(5):379-386.
23. Boissy A, Windover AK, Bokar D, et al. Communication skills training for physicians improves patient satisfaction. *J Gen Intern Med*. 2016;31(7):755-761.
24. Mougalian SS, Lessen DS, Levine RL, et al. Palliative care training and associations with burnout in oncology fellows. *J Support Oncol*. 2013;11(2):95-102.
25. Dwamena F, Holmes-Rovner M, Gaulden CM, et al. Interventions for providers to promote a patient-centred approach in clinical consultations. *Cochrane Database Syst Rev*. 2012;12:Cd003267.
26. Swayden KJ, Anderson KK, Connelly LM, Moran JS, McMahon JK, Arnold PM. Effect of sitting vs. standing on perception of provider time at bedside: a pilot study. *Patient Educ Couns*. 2012;86(2):166-171.
27. Tierney WM, Dexter PR, Gramelspacher GP, Perkins AJ, Zhou XH, Wolinsky FD. The effect of discussions about advance directives on patients' satisfaction with primary care. *J Gen Intern Med*. 2001;16(1):32-40.
28. Keating NL, Gandhi TK, Orav EJ, Bates DW, Ayanian JZ. Patient characteristics and experiences associated with trust in specialist physicians. *Arch Intern Med*. 2004;164(9):1015-1020.
29. Casarett D, Pickard A, Fishman JM, et al. Can metaphors and analogies improve communication with seriously ill patients? *J Palliat Med*. 2010;13(3):255-260.
30. McDonagh JR, Elliott TB, Engelberg RA, et al. Family satisfaction with family conferences about end-of-life care in the intensive care unit: increased proportion of family speech is associated with increased satisfaction. *Crit Care Med*. 2004;32(7):1484-1488.
31. Stapleton RD, Engelberg RA, Wenrich MD, Goss CH, Curtis JR. Clinician statements and family satisfaction with family conferences in the intensive care unit. *Crit Care Med*. 2006;34(6):1679-1685.
32. Heyland DK, Cook DJ, Rocker GM, et al. Decision-making in the ICU: perspectives of the substitute decision-maker. *Intensive Care Med*. 2003;29(1):75-82.
33. Tulsky JA. Beyond advance directives: importance of communication skills at the end of life. *JAMA*. 2005;294(3):359-365.
34. National Consensus Project for Quality Palliative Care. Clinical Practice Guidelines for Quality Palliative Care. 2nd ed. Pittsburgh, PA: National Consensus Project for Quality Palliative Care; 2009. http://www.nationalconsensusproject.org/guideline.pdf. Accessed April 28, 2017.
35. Institute of Medicine. Dying in America: Improving Quality and Honoring Individual Preferences Near the End of Life. Washington, DC: The National Academies Press; 2015. https://www.nap.edu/read/18748/chapter/1. Accessed April 28, 2017.
36. Del Vecchio Good MJ, Gadmer NM, Ruopp P, et al. Narrative nuances on good and bad deaths: internists' tales from high-technology work places. *Soc Sci Med*. 2004;58(5):939-953.
37. Weiner JS, Arnold RM, Curtis JR, Back AL, Rounsaville B, Tulsky JA. Manualized communication interventions to enhance palliative care research and training: rigorous, testable approaches. *J Palliat Med*. 2006;9(2):371-381.

38. Lorenz KA, Lynn J, Dy SM, et al. Cancer Care Quality Measures: Symptoms and End-of-Life Care. Rockville, MD: Agency for Healthcare Research and Quality. AHRQ Publication No. 06-E001; 2006. https://archive.ahrq.gov/downloads/pub/evidence/pdf/eolcanqm/eolcanqm.pdf. Accessed April 28, 2017.
39. Clarke EB, Curtis JR, Luce JM, et al. Quality indicators for end-of-life care in the intensive care unit. *Crit Care Med*. 2003;31(9):2255-2262.
40. Nelson JE, Mulkerin CM, Adams LL, Pronovost PJ. Improving comfort and communication in the ICU: a practical new tool for palliative care performance measurement and feedback. *Qual Saf Health Care*. 2006;15(4):264-271.
41. Visser M, Deliens L, Houttekier D. Physician-related barriers to communication and patient- and family-centred decision-making towards the end of life in intensive care: a systematic review. *Crit Care*. 2014;18(6):604.
42. NQF Endorses Palliative and End-of-Life Care Measures [press release]. Washington, DC: National Quality Forum; Feb 14, 2012. https://www.qualityforum.org/News_And_Resources/Press_Releases/2012/NQF_Endorses_Palliative_and_End-of-Life_Care_Measures.aspx. Accessed April 28, 2017.
43. Dy SM, Kiley KB, Ast K, et al. Measuring what matters: top-ranked quality indicators for hospice and palliative care from the American Academy of Hospice and Palliative Medicine and Hospice and Palliative Nurses Association. *J Pain Symptom Manage*. 2015;49(4):773-781.
44. Charon R. The patient-physician relationship. Narrative medicine: a model for empathy, reflection, profession, and trust. *JAMA*. 2001;286(15):1897-1902.
45. Weissman DE. Decision making at a time of crisis near the end of life. *JAMA*. 2004;292(14):1738-1743.
46. Buckman R. Communication in palliative care: a practical guide. In: Doyle D, Hanks GWC, MacDonald N, eds. *Oxford Textbook of Palliative Medicine*. 2nd ed. New York, NY: Oxford University Press; 1998:141-156.
47. Kon AA. The shared decision-making continuum. *JAMA*. 2010;304(8):903-904.
48. Ong LM, de Haes JC, Hoos AM, Lammes FB. Doctor-patient communication: a review of the literature. *Soc Sci Med*. 1995;40(7):903-918.
49. Jonsen AR, Siegler M, Winslade WJ. Clinical Ethics: A Practical Approach to Ethical Decisions in Clinical Medicine. 6th ed. New York, NY: Macmillan; 2006.
50. Quill TE. Perspectives on care at the close of life. Initiating end-of-life discussions with seriously ill patients: addressing the "elephant in the room". *JAMA*. 2000;284(19):2502-2507.
51. Lo B, Quill T, Tulsky J. Discussing palliative care with patients. ACP-ASIM End-of-Life Care Consensus Panel. American College of Physicians-American Society of Internal Medicine. *Ann Intern Med*. 1999;130(9):744-749.
52. von Gunten CF, Ferris FD, Emanuel LL. The patient-physician relationship. Ensuring competency in end-of-life care: communication and relational skills. *JAMA*. 2000;284(23):3051-3057.
53. Doukas DJ, Brody H. Care at the twilight: ethics and end-of-life care. *Am Fam Physician*. 1995;52(5):1294.
54. Doyle D. Have we looked beyond the physical and psychosocial? *J Pain Symptom Manage*. 1991;7(5):302-311.
55. Adson MA. An endangered ethic—the capacity for caring. *Mayo Clin Proc*. 1995;70(5):495-500.
56. Schweizer H. To give suffering a language. *Lit Med*. 1995;14(2):210-221.
57. Chaitchik S, Kreitler S, Shaked S, Schwartz I, Rosin R. Doctor-patient communication in a cancer ward. *J Cancer Educ*. 1992;7(1):41.
58. Knauft E, Nielsen EL, Engelberg RA, Patrick DL, Curtis JR. Barriers and facilitators to end-of-life care communication for patients with COPD. *Chest*. 2005;127(6):2188-2196.
59. Buckman R, Kason Y. *How to Break Bad News: A Guide for Health Care Professionals*. Baltimore, MD: Johns Hopkins University Press; 1992.
60. Holland JC, Almanza J. Giving bad news. Is there a kinder, gentler way? *Cancer*. 1999;86(5):738-740.

61. Ting-Toomey S. Communicating Across Cultures: The Guilford Communication Series. Guilford Press; 1999.
62. Lipson JG, Dibble SL, Minarik PA, eds. *Culture and Nursing Care: A Pocket Guide.* San Francisco, CA: UCSF Nursing Press; 1996.
63. Shrank WH, Kutner JS, Richardson T, Mularski RA, Fischer S, Kagawa-Singer M. Focus group findings about the influence of culture on communication preferences in end-of-life care. *J Gen Intern Med.* 2005;20(8):703-709.
64. Periyakoil VS, Neri E, Kraemer H. No easy talk: a mixed methods study of doctor reported barriers to conducting effective end-of-life conversations with diverse patients. *PLoS One.* 2015;10(4):e0122321.
65. Honeybun J, Johnston M, Tookman A. The impact of a death on fellow hospice patients. *Br J Med Psychol.* 1992;65:67-72.
66. Robinson TM, Alexander SC, Hays M, et al. Patient-oncologist communication in advanced cancer: predictors of patient perception of prognosis. *Support Care Cancer.* 2008;16(9):1049-1057.
67. Bruera E, Neumann CM, Mazzocato C, Stiefel F, Sala R. Attitudes and beliefs of palliative care physicians regarding communication with terminally ill cancer patients. *Palliat Med.* 2000;14(4):287-298.
68. Fitch MI. How much should I say to whom? *J Palliat Care.* 1994;10(3):90-100.
69. Kirk P, Kirk I, Kristjanson LJ. What do patients receiving palliative care for cancer and their families want to be told? A Canadian and Australian qualitative study. *BMJ.* 2004;328(7452):1343.
70. Voorhees J, Rietjens J, Onwuteaka-Philipsen B, et al. Discussing prognosis with terminally ill cancer patients and relatives: a survey of physicians' intentions in seven countries. *Patient Educ Couns.* 2009;77(3):430-436.
71. Vanchieri C. Cultural gaps leave patients angry, doctors confused. *J Natl Cancer Inst.* 1995;87(21):1576-1577.
72. Blackhall LJ, Murphy ST, Frank G, Michel V, Azen SP. Ethnicity and attitudes towards life sustaining technology. *JAMA.* 1995;274(10):820-825.
73. Morrison RS, Zayas LH, Mulvihill M, Baskin SA, Meier DE. Barriers to completion of health care proxies: an examination of ethnic differences. *Arch Intern Med.* 1998;158(22):2493-2497.
74. Kagawa-Singer M, Blackhall LJ. Negotiating cross-cultural issues at the end of life: "You got to go where he lives". *JAMA.* 2001;286(23):2993-3001.
75. Steinhauser KE, Voils CI, Clipp EC, Bosworth HB, Christakis NA, Tulsky JA. "Are you at peace?" One item to probe spiritual concerns at the end of life. *Arch Intern Med.* 2006;166(1):101-105.
76. Yardley SJ, Walshe CE, Parr A. Improving training in spiritual care: a qualitative study exploring patient perceptions of professional educational requirements. *Palliat Med.* 2009;23(7):601-607.
77. Hudson PL, Kristjanson LJ, Ashby M, et al. Desire for hastened death in patients with advanced disease and the evidence base of clinical guidelines: a systematic review. *Palliat Med.* 2006;20(7):693-701.
78. Oregon Public Health Division. Oregon Death with Dignity Act: 2015 Data Summary. Portland, OR: Oregon Health Authority; 2016. https://public.health.oregon.gov/ProviderPartnerResources/EvaluationResearch/DeathwithDignityAct/Documents/year18.pdf. Accessed April 28, 2017.
79. Solomon BK, Wilson KG, Henderson PR, Poulin PA, Kowal J, McKim DA. Loss of dignity in severe chronic obstructive pulmonary disease. *J Pain Symptom Manage.* 2016;51(3):529-537.
80. Lo C, Hales S, Jung J, et al. Managing Cancer And Living Meaningfully (CALM): phase 2 trial of a brief individual psychotherapy for patients with advanced cancer. *Palliat Med.* 2014;28(3):234-242.
81. Breitbart W, Rosenfeld B, Pessin H, Applebaum A, Kulikowski J, Lichtenthal WG. Meaning-centered group psychotherapy: an effective intervention for improving psychological well-being in patients with advanced cancer. *J Clin Oncol.* 2015;33(7):749-754.

82. A controlled trial to improve care for seriously ill hospitalized patients. The study to understand prognoses and preferences for outcomes and risks of treatments (SUPPORT). The SUPPORT Principal Investigators. *JAMA*. 1995;274(20):1591-1598.
83. Farber SJ, Egnew TR, Herman-Bertsch JL, Taylor TR, Guldin GE. Issues in end-of-life care: patient, caregiver, and clinician perceptions. *J Palliat Med*. 2003;6(1):19-31.
84. Rogers CR, Roethlisberger FJ. Barriers and gateways to communication. *Harv Bus Rev*. 1993;November/December:105-111.
85. Meier DE, Back AL, Morrison RS. The inner life of physicians and care of the seriously ill. *JAMA*. 2001;286(23):3007-3014.
86. Dosanjh S, Barnes J, Bhandari M. Barriers to breaking bad news among medical and surgical residents. *Med Educ*. 2001;35(3):197-205.
87. Baile WF, Lenzi R, Parker PA, Buckman R, Cohen L. Oncologists' attitudes toward and practices in giving bad news: an exploratory study. *J Clin Oncol*. 2002;20(8):2189-2196.
88. Bennett M, Alison D. Discussing the diagnosis and prognosis with cancer patients. *Postgrad Med J*. 1996;72(843):25-29.
89. Quill TE. Recognizing and adjusting to barriers in doctor-patient communication. *Ann Intern Med*. 1989;111(1):51-57.
90. Gattellari M, Voigt KJ, Butow PN, Tattersall MH. When the treatment goal is not cure: are cancer patients equipped to make informed decisions? *J Clin Oncol*. 2002;20(2):503-513.
91. Wright AA, Zhang B, Ray A, et al. Associations between end-of-life discussions, patient mental health, medical care near death, and caregiver bereavement adjustment. *JAMA*. 2008;300(14):1665-1673.
92. Mack JW, Block SD, Nilsson M, et al. Measuring therapeutic alliance between oncologists and patients with advanced cancer: the Human Connection Scale. *Cancer*. 2009;115(14):3302-3311.
93. Davison SN, Simpson C. Hope and advance care planning in patients with end stage renal disease: qualitative interview study. *BMJ*. 2006;333(7574):886.
94. Feifel H. Toward death: a psychological perspective. In: Schneidmen ES, ed. *Death: Current Perspectives*. Palo Alto, CA: Mayfield Publishing; 1976.
95. Granek L, Krzyzanowska MK, Tozer R, Mazzotta P. Oncologists' strategies and barriers to effective communication about the end of life. *J Oncol Pract*. 2013;9(4):e129-135.
96. Maguire P, Faulkner A. Improve the counselling skills of doctors and nurses in cancer care. *Br Med J*. 1988;297(6652):847-849.
97. White WL, Kunz C, Hogan J. Communication skills. *Hospice Education Program for Nurses*. Washington, DC: US Dept of Health and Human Services publication no. HRA 81-27; 1981.
98. Stone D, Patton B, Heen S. *Difficult Conversations*. 1st ed. New York, NY: Penguin Books; 2000.
99. Epstein RM. Mindful practice. *JAMA*. 1999;282(9):833-839.
100. Smith AK, Ritchie CS, Wallhagen ML. Hearing loss in hospice and palliative care: a national survey of providers. *J Pain Symptom Manage*. 2016;52(2):254-258.
101. Fogarty LA, Curbow BA, Wingard JR, McDonnell K, Somerfield MR. Can 40 seconds of compassion reduce patient anxiety? *J Clin Oncol*. 1999;17(1):371-379.
102. Levinson W, Gorawara-Bhat R, Lamb J. A study of patient clues and physician responses in primary care and surgical settings. *JAMA*. 2000;284(8):1021-1027.
103. Burgio KL, Williams BR, Dionne-Odom JN, et al. Racial differences in processes of care at end of life in VA medical centers: planned secondary analysis of data from the BEACON trial. *J Palliat Med*. 2016;19(2):157-163.
104. Johnson KS, Kuchibhatla M, Tulsky JA. Racial differences in self-reported exposure to information about hospice care. *J Palliat Med*. 2009;12(10):921-927.

105. Hadlow J, Pitts M. The understanding of common health terms by doctors, nurses and patients. *Soc Sci Med.* 1991;32(2):193-196.
106. Lichstein PR. The medical interview. In: Walker HK, Hall WD, Hurst JW, eds. *Clinical Methods: The History, Physical, and Laboratory Examinations.* 3rd ed. Boston, MA: Butterworths; 1990.
107. McCallister JW, Gustin JL, Wells-Di Gregorio S, Way DP, Mastronarde JG. Communication skills training curriculum for pulmonary and critical care fellows. *Ann Am Thorac Soc.* 2015;12(4):520-525.
108. Hope AA, Hsieh SJ, Howes JM, et al. Let's talk critical. Development and evaluation of a communication skills training program for critical care fellows. *Ann Am Thorac Soc.* 2015;12(4):505-511.
109. Arnold RM, Back AL, Barnato AE, et al. The Critical Care Communication project: improving fellows' communication skills. *J Crit Care.* 2015;30(2):250-254.
110. Kelley AS, Back AL, Arnold RM, et al. Geritalk: communication skills training for geriatric and palliative medicine fellows. *J Am Geriatr Soc.* 2012;60(2):332-337.
111. Bensing J. Doctor-patient communication and the quality of care. *Soc Sci Med.* 1991;32(11):1301-1310.
112. Friedman HS. Non-verbal communications between patients and medical practitioners. *J Soc Issues.* 1979;35:82.
113. Lumsden G, Lumsden DL. *Communicating in Groups and Teams: Sharing Leadership.* 4th ed. Belmont, CA: Thomson/Wadsworth; 2004.
114. Back AL, Anderson WG, Bunch L, et al. Communication about cancer near the end of life. *Cancer.* 2008;113(7 Suppl):1897-1910.
115. Hamilton C, Parker C. Communicating for Results: A Guide for Business and the Professions. 4th ed. Belmont, CA: Wadsworth; 1993.
116. Delbanco TL. Enriching the doctor-patient relationship by inviting the patient's perspective. *Ann Intern Med.* 1992;116(5):414-418.
117. Miller RJ. Communication and truth telling in terminal illness. Academy of Hospice Physicians Annual Assembly; April, 1992; Philadelphia, PA.
118. Marvel MK, Epstein RM, Flowers K, Beckman HB. Soliciting the patient's agenda: have we improved? *JAMA.* 1999;281(3):283-287.
119. Kleinman A. The Illness Narratives: Suffering, Healing and the Human Condition. New York, NY: Basic Books, Inc.; 1998.
120. Chochinov HM, Hack T, Hassard T, Kristjanson LJ, McClement S, Harlos M. Dignity therapy: a novel psychotherapeutic intervention for patients near the end of life. *J Clin Oncol.* 2005;23(24):5520-5525.
121. Chochinov HM, Kristjanson LJ, Breitbart W, et al. Effect of dignity therapy on distress and end-of-life experience in terminally ill patients: a randomised controlled trial. *Lancet Oncol.* 2011;12(8):753-762.
122. Williamson DS, Noel ML. Systemic family medicine: an evolving concept. In: Rakel RE, ed. *Textbook of Family Practice.* 4th ed. Philadelphia, PA: WB Saunders; 1990:61-79.
123. Back AL, Arnold RM, Baile WF, Tulsky JA, Fryer-Edwards K. Approaching difficult communication tasks in oncology. *CA Cancer J Clin.* 2005;55(3):164-177.
124. Wittenberg E, Ferrell B, Goldsmith J, et al., eds. *Textbook of Palliative Care Communication.* New York, NY: Oxford University Press; 2015.
125. Lunn L. Spritual concerns in palliation. In: Saunders C, Sykes N, eds. *Management of Terminal Malignancies.* 3rd ed. Boston, MA: Edward Arnold; 1993.
126. Ptacek JT, Eberhardt TL. Breaking bad news. A review of the literature. *JAMA.* 1996;276(6):496-502.
127. Selph RB, Shiang J, Engelberg R, Curtis JR, White DB. Empathy and life support decisions in intensive care units. *J Gen Intern Med.* 2008;23(9):1311-1317.

128. Pollak KI, Arnold R, Alexander SC, et al. Do patient attributes predict oncologist empathic responses and patient perceptions of empathy? *Support Care Cancer.* 2010;18(11):1405-1411.
129. Pollak KI, Arnold RM, Jeffreys AS, et al. Oncologist communication about emotion during visits with patients with advanced cancer. *J Clin Oncol.* 2007;25(36):5748-5752.
130. Kennifer SL, Alexander SC, Pollak KI, et al. Negative emotions in cancer care: do oncologists' responses depend on severity and type of emotion? *Patient Educ Couns.* 2009;76(1):51-56.
131. Jansen J, van Weert JC, de Groot J, van Dulmen S, Heeren TJ, Bensing JM. Emotional and informational patient cues: the impact of nurses' responses on recall. *Patient Educ Couns.* 2010;79(2):218-224.
132. Morgan PA, de Oliveira JS, Alexander SC, et al. Comparing oncologist, nurse, and physician assistant attitudes toward discussions of negative emotions with patients. *J Physician Assist Educ.* 2010;21(3):13-17.
133. Johnson RF, Jr., Gustin J. Acute lung injury and acute respiratory distress syndrome requiring tracheal intubation and mechanical ventilation in the intensive care unit: impact on managing uncertainty for patient-centered communication. *Am J Hosp Palliat Care.* 2013;30(6):569-575.
134. Dean RA. Humor and laughter in palliative care. *J Palliat Care.* 1997;13(1):34-39.
135. Fry WF, Jr. The physiologic effects of humor, mirth, and laughter. *JAMA.* 1992;267(13):1857-1858.
136. Wooten P. Humor: an antidote for stress. *Holist Nurs Pract.* 1996;10(2):49-56.
137. Steinhauser KE, Christakis NA, Clipp EC, McNeilly M, McIntyre L, Tulsky JA. Factors considered important at the end of life by patients, family, physicians, and other care providers. *JAMA.* 2000;284(19):2476-2482.
138. Ridley J, Dance D, Pare D. The acceptability of humor between palliative care patients and health care providers. *J Palliat Med.* 2014;17(4):472-474.
139. Goodman JB. Laughing matters: taking your job seriously and yourself lightly. *JAMA.* 1992;267(13):1858.
140. Perrino AF. *Holyquest: The Search for Wholeness.* Carmel, CA: Sunflower Ink; 1988.
141. Herth K. Fostering hope in terminally ill people. *J Adv Nurs.* 1990;15(11):1250-1259.
142. Johnston M, Earll L, Mitchell E, Morrison V, Wright S. Communicating the diagnosis of motor neurone disease. *Palliat Med.* 1996;10(1):23-34.
143. Morita T, Akechi T, Ikenaga M, et al. Communication about the ending of anticancer treatment and transition to palliative care. *Ann Oncol.* 2004;15(10):1551-1557.
144. Robinson I. *Multiple Sclerosis (Experience of Illness).* London: Routledge; 1988.
145. Foley K. A 44-year-old woman with severe pain at the end of life. *JAMA.* 1999;281(20):1937-1945.
146. von Gunten CF. Discussing hospice care. *J Clin Oncol.* 2002;20(5):1419-1424.
147. Bousquet G, Orri M, Winterman S, Brugiere C, Verneuil L, Revah-Levy A. Breaking bad news in oncology: A metasynthesis. *J Clin Oncol.* 2015;33(22):2437-2443.
148. Back AL, Trinidad SB, Hopley EK, Arnold RM, Baile WF, Edwards KA. What patients value when oncologists give news of cancer recurrence: commentary on specific moments in audio-recorded conversations. *Oncologist.* 2011;16(3):342-350.
149. Baile WF, Buckman R, Lenzi R, Glober G, Beale EA, Kudelka AP. SPIKES-A six-step protocol for delivering bad news: application to the patient with cancer. *Oncologist.* 2000;5(4):302-311.
150. Fallowfield L, Jenkins V. Communicating sad, bad, and difficult news in medicine. *Lancet.* 2004;363(9405):312-319.
151. Rabow MW, McPhee SJ. Beyond breaking bad news: how to help patients who suffer. *West J Med.* 1999;171(4):260-263.
152. Baile WF, Buckman R, Lenzi R, Glober G, Beale EA, Kudelka AP. SPIKES—A six-step protocol for delivering bad news: application to the patient with cancer. *Oncologist.* 2000;5(4):302-311.

153. Clayton JM, Butow PN, Tattersall MH. When and how to initiate discussion about prognosis and end-of-life issues with terminally ill patients. *J Pain Symptom Manage.* 2005;30(2):132-144.
154. O'Toole E, Step MM, Engelhardt K, Lewis S, Rose JH. The role of primary care physicians in advanced cancer care: perspectives of older patients and their oncologists. *J Am Geriatr Soc.* 2009;57 Suppl 2:S265-268.
155. Repetto L, Piselli P, Raffaele M, Locatelli C. Communicating cancer diagnosis and prognosis: when the target is the elderly patient-a GIOGer study. *Eur J Cancer.* 2009;45(3):374-383.
156. Fukui S, Ogawa K, Ohtsuka M, Fukui N. A randomized study assessing the efficacy of communication skill training on patients' psychologic distress and coping: nurses' communication with patients just after being diagnosed with cancer. *Cancer.* 2008;113(6):1462-1470.
157. Bruera E, Palmer JL, Pace E, et al. A randomized, controlled trial of physician postures when breaking bad news to cancer patients. *Palliat Med.* 2007;21(6):501-505.
158. Waitzkin H. Doctor-patient communication. Clinical implications of social scientific research. *JAMA.* 1984;252(17):2441-2446. Soc Sci Med.
159. Hanratty B, Lowson E, Holmes L, et al. Breaking bad news sensitively: what is important to patients in their last year of life? *BMJ Support Palliat Care.* 2012;2(1):24-28.
160. Lagarde SM, Franssen SJ, van Werven JR, et al. Patient preferences for the disclosure of prognosis after esophagectomy for cancer with curative intent. *Ann Surg Oncol.* 2008;15(11):3289-3298.
161. Apatira L, Boyd EA, Malvar G, et al. Hope, truth, and preparing for death: perspectives of surrogate decision makers. *Ann Intern Med.* 2008;149(12):861-868.
162. Alexander SC, Ladwig S, Norton SA, et al. Emotional distress and compassionate responses in palliative care decision-making consultations. *J Palliat Med.* 2014;17(5):579-584.
163. Sep MS, van Osch M, van Vliet LM, Smets EM, Bensing JM. The power of clinicians' affective communication: how reassurance about non-abandonment can reduce patients' physiological arousal and increase information recall in bad news consultations. An experimental study using analogue patients. *Patient Educ Couns.* 2014;95(1):45-52.
164. Ford S, Fallowfield L, Lewis S. Can oncologists detect distress in their out-patients and how satisfied are they with their performance during bad news consultations? *Br J Cancer.* 1994;70(4):767-770.
165. Merckaert I, Libert Y, Delvaux N, et al. Factors that influence physicians' detection of distress in patients with cancer: can a communication skills training program improve physicians' detection? *Cancer.* 2005;104(2):411-421.
166. Campbell TC, Carey EC, Jackson VA, et al. Discussing prognosis: balancing hope and realism. *Cancer J.* 2010;16(5):461-466.
167. Windover A, Boissy A, Rice TW, Merlino J, Gilligan T, Velez V. The REDE model of healthcare communication: Optimizing relationship as a therapeutic agent. *J Patient Exper.* 2014;1(1):8-13.
168. Fallowfield L. Giving sad and bad news. *Lancet.* 1993;341(8843):476-478.
169. O'Grady E, Dempsey L, Fabby C. Anger: a common form of psychological distress among patients at the end of life. *Int J Palliat Nurs.* 2012;18(12):592-596.
170. Quill TE, Arnold RM, Platt F. "I wish things were different": expressing wishes in response to loss, futility, and unrealistic hopes. *Ann Intern Med.* 2001;135(7):551-555.
171. Back AL, Arnold RM. "Yes it's sad, but what should I do?" Moving from empathy to action in discussing goals of care. *J Palliat Med.* 2014;17(2):141-144.
172. Back AL, Arnold RM, Quill TE. Hope for the best, and prepare for the worst. *Ann Intern Med.* 2003;138(5):439-443.
173. Roe E. Practical strategies for death notification in the emergency department. *J Emerg Nurs.* 2012;38(2):130-134; quiz 200.

174. Taylor E. How best to communicate bad news over the telephone. *End of Life Care*. 2007;1(1). http://eolj.bmj.com/content/eolcare/1/1/30. Accessed July 3, 2017.
175. Rosenbaum GE, Burns J, Johnson J, Mitchell C, Robinson M, Truog RD. Autopsy consent practice at US teaching hospitals: results of a national survey. *Arch Intern Med*. 2000;160(3):374-380.
176. Rokoske FS, Schenck AP, Hanson LC. The potential use of autopsy for continuous quality improvement in hospice and palliative care. *Medscape J Med*. 2008;10(12):289.
177. Billings JA, Krakauer EL. On patient autonomy and physician responsibility in end-of-life care. *Arch Intern Med*. 2011;171(9):849-853.
178. Billings JA. The end-of-life family meeting in intensive care part II: Family-centered decision making. *J Palliat Med*. 2011;14(9):1051-1057.
179. VitalTalk. Addressing goals of care: "REMAP". http://www.vitaltalk.org/quick-guides. Accessed April 24, 2017.
180. Jackson VA, Jacobsen J, Greer JA, Pirl WF, Temel JS, Back AL. The cultivation of prognostic awareness through the provision of early palliative care in the ambulatory setting: a communication guide. *J Palliat Med*. 2013;16(8):894-900.
181. Quill TE, Brody H. Physician recommendations and patient autonomy: finding a balance between physician power and patient choice. *Ann Intern Med*. 1996;125(9):763-769.
182. Roeland E, Cain J, Onderdonk C, Kerr K, Mitchell W, Thornberry K. When open-ended questions don't work: the role of palliative paternalism in difficult medical decisions. *J Palliat Med*. 2014;17(4):415-420.
183. Gawande A. *Being Mortal*. New York: Metropolitan Books, Henry Holt and Company; 2014.
184. Curtis JR, Engelberg RA, Nielsen EL, Au DH, Patrick DL. Patient-physician communication about end-of-life care for patients with severe COPD. *Eur Respir J*. 2004;24(2):200-205.
185. Koedoot CG, Oort FJ, de Haan RJ, Bakker PJ, de Graeff A, de Haes JC. The content and amount of information given by medical oncologists when telling patients with advanced cancer what their treatment options are. Palliative chemotherapy and watchful-waiting. *Eur J Cancer*. 2004;40(2):225-235.
186. White DB, Engelberg RA, Wenrich MD, Lo B, Curtis JR. Prognostication during physician-family discussions about limiting life support in intensive care units. *Crit Care Med*. 2007;35(2):442-448.
187. Christakis NA, Lamont EB. Extent and determinants of error in doctors' prognoses in terminally ill patients: prospective cohort study. *BMJ*. 2000;320(7233):469-472.
188. Lamont EB, Christakis NA. Prognostic disclosure to patients with cancer near the end of life. *Ann Intern Med*. 2001;134(12):1096-1105.
189. Harding R, Selman L, Beynon T, et al. Meeting the communication and information needs of chronic heart failure patients. *J Pain Symptom Manage*. 2008;36(2):149-156.
190. Jenkins V, Solis-Trapala I, Langridge C, Catt S, Talbot DC, Fallowfield LJ. What oncologists believe they said and what patients believe they heard: an analysis of phase I trial discussions. *J Clin Oncol*. 2011;29(1):61-68.
191. Audrey S, Abel J, Blazeby JM, Falk S, Campbell R. What oncologists tell patients about survival benefits of palliative chemotherapy and implications for informed consent: qualitative study. *BMJ*. 2008;337:a752.
192. Rodriguez KL, Gambino FJ, Butow PN, Hagerty RG, Arnold RM. 'It's going to shorten your life': framing of oncologist-patient communication about prognosis. *Psychooncology*. 2008;17(3):219-225.
193. Keating NL, Landrum MB, Rogers SO, Jr., et al. Physician factors associated with discussions about end-of-life care. *Cancer*. 2010;116(4):998-1006.
194. White DB, Engelberg RA, Wenrich MD, Lo B, Curtis JR. The language of prognostication in intensive care units. *Med Decis Making*. 2010;30(1):76-83.
195. Tanco K, Rhondali W, Perez-Cruz P, et al. Patient perception of physician compassion after a more optimistic vs a less optimistic message: a randomized clinical trial. *JAMA Oncol*. 2015;1(2):176-183.

196. Hagerty RG, Butow PN, Ellis PM, et al. Communicating with realism and hope: incurable cancer patients' views on the disclosure of prognosis. *J Clin Oncol.* 2005;23(6):1278-1288.
197. Weeks JC, Cook EF, O'Day SJ, et al. Relationship between cancer patients' predictions of prognosis and their treatment preferences. *JAMA.* 1998;279(21):1709-1714.
198. Murphy DJ, Burrows D, Santilli S, et al. The influence of the probability of survival on patients' preferences regarding cardiopulmonary resuscitation. *N Engl J Med.* 1994;330(8):545-549.
199. Wagner GJ, Riopelle D, Steckart J, Lorenz KA, Rosenfeld KE. Provider communication and patient understanding of life-limiting illness and their relationship to patient communication of treatment preferences. *J Pain Symptom Manage.* 2010;39(3):527-534.
200. Zier LS, Burack JH, Micco G, et al. Doubt and belief in physicians' ability to prognosticate during critical illness: the perspective of surrogate decision makers. *Crit Care Med.* 2008;36(8):2341-2347.
201. Boyd EA, Lo B, Evans LR, et al. "It's not just what the doctor tells me:" factors that influence surrogate decision-makers' perceptions of prognosis. *Crit Care Med.* 2010;38(5):1270-1275.
202. Hagerty RG, Butow PN, Ellis PA, et al. Cancer patient preferences for communication of prognosis in the metastatic setting. *J Clin Oncol.* 2004;22(9):1721-1730.
203. Pfeifer MP, Mitchell CK, Chamberlain L. The value of disease severity in predicting patient readiness to address end-of-life issues. *Arch Intern Med.* 2003;163(5):609-612.
204. Back AL, Arnold RM. Discussing prognosis: "How much do you want to know?" Talking to patients who are prepared for explicit information. *J Clin Oncol.* 2006;24(25):4209-4213.
205. Allen LA, Yager JE, Funk MJ, et al. Discordance between patient-predicted and model-predicted life expectancy among ambulatory patients with heart failure. *JAMA.* 2008;299(21):2533-2542.
206. Patel D, Cohen ED, Barnato AE. The effect of framing on surrogate optimism bias: a simulation study. *J Crit Care.* 2016;32:85-88.
207. Butow PN, Dowsett S, Hagerty R, Tattersall MH. Communicating prognosis to patients with metastatic disease: what do they really want to know? *Support Care Cancer.* 2002;10(2):161-168.
208. Lee Char SJ, Evans LR, Malvar GL, White DB. A randomized trial of two methods to disclose prognosis to surrogate decision makers in intensive care units. *Am J Respir Crit Care Med.* 2010;182(7):905-909.
209. Gordon GH, Joos SK, Byrne J. Physician expressions of uncertainty during patient encounters. *Patient Educ Couns.* 2000;40(1):59-65.
210. Evans LR, Boyd EA, Malvar G, et al. Surrogate decision-makers' perspectives on discussing prognosis in the face of uncertainty. *Am J Respir Crit Care Med.* 2009;179(1):48-53.
211. Hebert RS, Schulz R, Copeland VC, Arnold RM. Preparing family caregivers for death and bereavement. Insights from caregivers of terminally ill patients. *J Pain Symptom Manage.* 2009;37(1):3-12.
212. Smith AK, White DB, Arnold RM. Uncertainty—the other side of prognosis. *N Engl J Med.* 2013;368(26):2448-2450.
213. Byock I. Dying Well: The Prospect for Growth at the End of Life. New York, NY: Riverhead; 1997.
214. Schonwetter RS, Teasdale TA, Storey P, Luchi RJ. Estimation of survival time in terminal cancer patients: an impedance to hospice admissions? *Hosp J.* 1990;6(4):65-79.
215. Krishnan MS, Epstein-Peterson Z, Chen YH, et al. Predicting life expectancy in patients with metastatic cancer receiving palliative radiotherapy: the TEACHH model. *Cancer.* 2014;120(1):134-141.
216. Vachon M. The emotional problems of the patient in palliative medicine. In: Hanks G, Cherny N, Christakis N, Fallon M, Kaasa S, Portenoy RK, eds. *Oxford Textbook of Palliaitve Medicine.* 4th ed. New York, NY: Oxford University Press; 2010:1410-1436.
217. Renz M, Mao MS, Bueche D, Cerny T, Strasser F. Dying is a transition. *Am J Hosp Palliat Care.* 2013;30(3):283-290.

218. Kogan NR, Dumas M, Cohen SR. The extra burdens patients in denial impose on their family caregivers. *Palliat Support Care*. 2013;11(2):91-99.
219. Cepeda MS, Chapman CR, Miranda N, et al. Emotional disclosure through patient narrative may improve pain and well-being: results of a randomized controlled trial in patients with cancer pain. *J Pain Symptom Manage*. 2008;35(6):623-631.
220. Moore RJ, Hallenbeck J. Narrative empathy and how dealing with stories helps: creating a space for empathy in culturally diverse care settings. *J Pain Symptom Manage*. 2010;40(3):471-476.
221. Chittem M, Butow P. Responding to family requests for nondisclosure: the impact of oncologists' cultural background. *J Cancer Res Ther*. 2015;11(1):174-180.
222. Hallenbeck J, Arnold R. A request for nondisclosure: don't tell mother. *J Clin Oncol*. 2007;25(31):5030-5034.
223. Giacalone A, Talamini R, Spina M, Fratino L, Spazzapan S, Tirelli U. Can the caregiver replace his/her elderly cancer patient in the physician-patient line of communication? *Support Care Cancer*. 2008;16(10):1157-1162.
224. Powazki R, Walsh D, Hauser K, Davis MP. Communication in palliative medicine: a clinical review of family conferences. *J Palliat Med*. 2014;17(10):1167-1177.
225. Lilly CM, Sonna LA, Haley KJ, Massaro AF. Intensive communication: four-year follow-up from a clinical practice study. *Crit Care Med*. 2003;31(5 Suppl):S394-399.
226. Lautrette A, Darmon M, Megarbane B, et al. A communication strategy and brochure for relatives of patients dying in the ICU. *N Engl J Med*. 2007;356(5):469-478.
227. Azoulay E, Pochard F. Communication with family members of patients dying in the intensive care unit. *Curr Opin Crit Care*. 2003;9(6):545-550.
228. Azoulay E, Pochard F, Kentish-Barnes N, et al. Risk of post-traumatic stress symptoms in family members of intensive care unit patients. *Am J Respir Crit Care Med*. 2005;171(9):987-994.
229. Minuchin S. *Families and Family Therapy*. Cambridge, MA: Harvard University Press; 1974.
230. Satir V. *The New Peoplemaking*. Mountain View, CA: Science and Behavior Books; 1988.
231. Nicholls D, Chang E, Johnson A, Edenborough M. Touch, the essence of caring for people with end-stage dementia: a mental health perspective in Namaste Care. *Aging Ment Health*. 2013;17(5):571-578.
232. De Vleminck A, Pardon K, Beernaert K, et al. Barriers to advance care planning in cancer, heart failure and dementia patients: a focus group study on general practitioners' views and experiences. *PLoS One*. 2014;9(1):e84905.
233. Cohen AB, Wright MS, Cooney L, Jr., Fried T. Guardianship and End-of-Life Decision Making. *JAMA Intern Med*. 2015;175(10):1687-1691.
234. Cohen S, Sprung C, Sjokvist P, et al. Communication of end-of-life decisions in European intensive care units. *Intensive Care Med*. 2005;31(9):1215-1221.
235. Gordon NP, Shade SB. Advance directives are more likely among seniors asked about end-of-life care preferences. *Arch Intern Med*. 1999;159(7):701-704.
236. Danis M, Southerland LI, Garrett JM, et al. A prospective study of advance directives for life-sustaining care. *N Engl J Med*. 1991;324(13):882-888.
237. Bakitas M, Ahles TA, Skalla K, et al. Proxy perspectives regarding end-of-life care for persons with cancer. *Cancer*. 2008;112(8):1854-1861.
238. Curtis JR, Patrick DL, Shannon SE, Treece PD, Engelberg RA, Rubenfeld GD. The family conference as a focus to improve communication about end-of-life care in the intensive care unit: opportunities for improvement. *Crit Care Med*. 2001;29(2 Suppl):26-33.
239. Lang F, Quill T. Making decisions with families at the end of life. *Am Fam Physician*. 2004;70(4):719-723.

240. Rabow MW, Hauser JM, Adams J. Supporting family caregivers at the end of life: "They don't know what they don't know". *JAMA.* 2004;291(4):483-491.
241. Nelson JE, Walker AS, Luhrs CA, Cortez TB, Pronovost PJ. Family meetings made simpler: a toolkit for the intensive care unit. *J Crit Care.* 2009;24(4):626 e627-614.
242. Seckler AB, Meier DE, Mulvihill M, Paris BE. Substituted judgment: how accurate are proxy predictions? *Ann Intern Med.* 1991;115(2):92-98.
243. Schenker Y, Crowley-Matoka M, Dohan D, Tiver GA, Arnold RM, White DB. I don't want to be the one saying 'we should just let him die': intrapersonal tensions experienced by surrogate decision makers in the ICU. *J Gen Intern Med.* 2012;27(12):1657-1665.
244. Gries CJ, Curtis JR, Wall RJ, Engelberg RA. Family member satisfaction with end-of-life decision making in the ICU. *Chest.* 2008;133(3):704-712.
245. White DB, Evans LR, Bautista CA, Luce JM, Lo B. Are physicians' recommendations to limit life support beneficial or burdensome? Bringing empirical data to the debate. *Am J Respir Crit Care Med.* 2009;180(4):320-325.
246. White DB, Malvar G, Karr J, Lo B, Curtis JR. Expanding the paradigm of the physician's role in surrogate decision-making: an empirically derived framework. *Crit Care Med.* 2010;38(3):743-750.
247. Gries CJ, Engelberg RA, Kross EK, et al. Predictors of symptoms of posttraumatic stress and depression in family members after patient death in the ICU. *Chest.* 2010;137(2):280-287.
248. Johnson SK, Bautista CA, Hong SY, Weissfeld L, White DB. An empirical study of surrogates' preferred level of control over value-laden life support decisions in intensive care units. *Am J Respir Crit Care Med.* 2011;183(7):915-921.
249. White DB, Braddock CH, 3rd, Bereknyei S, Curtis JR. Toward shared decision making at the end of life in intensive care units: opportunities for improvement. *Arch Intern Med.* 2007;167(5):461-467.
250. Norton SA, Metzger M, DeLuca J, Alexander SC, Quill TE, Gramling R. Palliative care communication: linking patients' prognoses, values, and goals of care. *Res Nurs Health.* 2013;36(6):582-590.
251. Karlawish JH, Quill T, Meier DE. A consensus-based approach to providing palliative care to patients who lack decision-making capacity. *Ann Intern Med.* 1999;130(10):835-840.
252. Miller JJ, Morris P, Files DC, Gower E, Young M. Decision conflict and regret among surrogate decision makers in the medical intensive care unit. *J Crit Care.* 2016;32:79-84.
253. Abbott KH, Sago JG, Breen CM, Abernethy AP, Tulsky JA. Families looking back: one year after discussion of withdrawal or withholding of life-sustaining support. *Crit Care Med.* 2001;29(1):197-201.
254. Burns JP, Mello MM, Studdert DM, Puopolo AL, Truog RD, Brennan TA. Results of a clinical trial on care improvement for the critically ill. *Crit Care Med.* 2003;31(8):2107-2117.
255. Quill TE, Arnold R, Back AL. Discussing treatment preferences with patients who want "everything". *Ann Intern Med.* 2009;151(5):345-349.
256. Puchalski C, Handzo G, Ferrell B. Religious conflicts: decision making when religious beliefs and medical realities conflict (P17). *J Pain Symptom Manage.* 2016;51(2):313-314.
257. Cooper RS, Ferguson A, Bodurtha JN, Smith TJ. AMEN in challenging conversations: bridging the gaps between faith, hope, and medicine. *J Oncol Pract.* 2014;10(4):e191-195.
258. Fisher R, Ury W. *Getting to Yes: Negotiating Agreement Without Giving In.* Boston, MA: Houghton-Mifflin; 1981.
259. Back AL, Arnold RM. Dealing with conflict in caring for the seriously ill: "it was just out of the question". *JAMA.* 2005;293(11):1374-1381.
260. Jimenez XF, Hernandez JO, Robinson EM. When mediation fails: identifying and working with inappropriate surrogate decision makers. *Prog Pall Care.* 2015;23(3):142-147.

261. Werth JL, Burke C, Bardash RJ. Confidentiality in end-of-life and after-death situations. *Ethics Behav.* 2002;12(3):205-222.
262. Baumrucker SJ, Carter GT, Adkins RW, et al. The deathbed confession. *Am J Hosp Palliat Care.* 2014;31(5):576-580.
263. Byock I, Palac D. Confidentiality. In: Hanks GWC, Cherny NI, Christakis NA, Fallon M, Kaasa S, Portenoy RK, eds. *Oxford Textbook of Palliative Medicine.* 4th ed. New York, NY: Oxford University Press; 2010:281-289.
264. Cheung W, Aggarwal G, Fugaccia E, et al. Palliative care teams in the intensive care unit: a randomised, controlled, feasibility study. *Crit Care Resusc.* 2010;12(1):28-35.
265. O'Mahony S, McHenry J, Blank AE, et al. Preliminary report of the integration of a palliative care team into an intensive care unit. *Palliat Med.* 2010;24(2):154-165.
266. Curtis JR, Treece PD, Nielsen EL, et al. Integrating palliative and critical care: evaluation of a quality-improvement intervention. *Am J Respir Crit Care Med.* 2008;178(3):269-275.
267. Norton SA, Hogan LA, Holloway RG, Temkin-Greener H, Buckley MJ, Quill TE. Proactive palliative care in the medical intensive care unit: effects on length of stay for selected high-risk patients. *Crit Care Med.* 2007;35(6):1530-1535.
268. Lawson BJ, Burge FI, McIntyre P, Field S, Maxwell D. Palliative care patients in the emergency department. *J Palliat Care.* 2008;24(4):247-255.
269. Le Conte P, Riochet D, Batard E, et al. Death in emergency departments: a multicenter cross-sectional survey with analysis of withholding and withdrawing life support. *Intensive Care Med.* 2010;36(5):765-772.
270. Wiese CH, Bartels UE, Marczynska K, Ruppert D, Graf BM, Hanekop GG. Quality of out-of-hospital palliative emergency care depends on the expertise of the emergency medical team—a prospective multi-centre analysis. *Support Care Cancer.* 2009;17(12):1499-1506.
271. George N, Phillips E, Zaurova M, Song C, Lamba S, Grudzen C. Palliative care screening and assessment in the emergency department: a systematic review. *J Pain Symptom Manage.* 2016;51(1):108-119.e102.
272. Palliative program yields triage changes in the ED. *ED Manag.* 2007;19(3):27-29.
273. Smith AK, Schonberg MA, Fisher J, et al. Emergency department experiences of acutely symptomatic patients with terminal illness and their family caregivers. *J Pain Symptom Manage.* 2010;39(6):972-981.
274. Smith AK, Fisher J, Schonberg MA, et al. Am I doing the right thing? Provider perspectives on improving palliative care in the emergency department. *Ann Emerg Med.* 2009;54(1):86-93, 93 e81.
275. Rocque GB, Campbell TC, Johnson SK, et al. A quantitative study of triggered palliative care consultation for hospitalized patients with advanced cancer. *J Pain Symptom Manage.* 2015;50(4):462-469.
276. Zalenski R, Courage C, Edelen A, et al. Evaluation of screening criteria for palliative care consultation in the MICU: a multihospital analysis. *BMJ Support Palliat Care.* 2014;4(3):254-262.
277. Meier DE, Beresford L. Consultation etiquette challenges palliative care to be on its best behavior. *J Palliat Med.* 2007;10(1):7-11.
278. Salerno SM, Hurst FP, Halvorson S, Mercado DL. Principles of effective consultation: an update for the 21st-century consultant. *Arch Intern Med.* 2007;167(3):271-275.
279. Goldman L, Lee T, Rudd P. Ten commandments for effective consultations. *Arch Intern Med.* 1983;143(9):1753-1755.
280. Kenen J. Palliative care in the emergency department: new specialty weaving into acute care fabric. *Ann Emerg Med.* 2010;56(6):A17-19.
281. Thurston A, Fettig L, Arnold R. Team communication in the acute care setting. *Textbook of Palliative Care Communication.* Oxford, UK: Oxford University Press; 2015:321-329.
282. Hurley AC, Volicer L. Alzheimer Disease: "It's okay, Mama, if you want to go, it's okay". *JAMA.* 2002;288(18):2324-2331.

283. Gessert CE, Forbes S, Bern-Klug M. Planning end-of-life care for patients with dementia: roles of families and health professionals. *Omega (Westport)*. 2000;42(4):273-291.
284. McCann RM, Hall WJ, Groth-Juncker A. Comfort care for terminally ill patients. The appropriate use of nutrition and hydration. *JAMA*. 1994;272(16):1263-1266.
285. Mitchell SL, Teno JM, Kiely DK, et al. The clinical course of advanced dementia. *N Engl J Med*. 2009;361(16):1529-1538.
286. Sampson EL, Candy B, Jones L. Enteral tube feeding for older people with advanced dementia. *Cochrane Database Syst Rev*. 2009(2):CD007209.
287. Kukull WA, Brenner DE, Speck CE, et al. Causes of death associated with Alzheimer disease: variation by level of cognitive impairment before death. *J Am Geriatr Soc*. 1994;42(7):723-726.
288. Givens JL, Jones RN, Shaffer ML, Kiely DK, Mitchell SL. Survival and comfort after treatment of pneumonia in advanced dementia. *Arch Intern Med*. 2010;170(13):1102-1107.
289. Albinsson L, Strang P. Differences in supporting families of dementia patients and cancer patients: a palliative perspective. *Palliat Med*. 2003;17(4):359-367.
290. Teno JM, Gozalo PL, Lee IC, et al. Does hospice improve quality of care for persons dying from dementia? *J Am Geriatr Soc*. 2011;59(8):1531-1536.
291. Thompson PM. Communicating with dementia patients on hospice. *Am J Hosp Palliat Care*. 2002;19(4):263-266.
292. Eggenberger E, Heimerl K, Bennett MI. Communication skills training in dementia care: a systematic review of effectiveness, training content, and didactic methods in different care settings. *Int Psychogeriatr*. 2013;25(3):345-358.
293. Zachariah F, Thomson B, Loscalzo M, Crocitto L. Care coordination and transitions in care. In: Wittenberg E, Ferrell BR, Goldsmith J, Smith T, Glajchen M, Handzo GF, eds. *Textbook of Palliative Care Communication*. New York, NY: Oxford University Press; 2015:246-254.
294. Christ GH, Christ AE. Current approaches to helping children cope with a parent's terminal illness. *CA Cancer J Clin*. 2006;56(4):197-212.
295. Rauch PK, Muriel AC, Cassem NH. Parents with cancer: who's looking after the children? *J Clin Oncol*. 2002;20(21):4399-4402.
296. Goldman A, Hain R, Liben S, eds. *Oxford Textbook of Palliative Care for Children*. 2nd ed. New York, NY: Oxford Univeristy Press; 2012.
297. Kircher PM. *Love Is the Link: A Hospice Doctor Shares Her Experience of Near-Death and Dying*. Burdett, NY: Larson Publications; 1995.
298. Callanan M, Kelley P. *Final Gifts: Understanding the Special Awareness, Needs, and Communications of the Dying*. New York, NY: Bantam; 1997.
299. Kerr CW, Donnelly JP, Wright ST, et al. End-of-life dreams and visions: a longitudinal study of hospice patients' experiences. *J Palliat Med*. 2014;17(3):296-303.
300. Engelberg RA, Wenrich MD, Curtis JR. Responding to families' questions about the meaning of physical movements in critically ill patients. *J Crit Care*. 2008;23(4):565-571.
301. American Telemedicine Association. What is telemedicine? 2012; http://www.americantelemed.org/about/telehealth-faqs. Accessed June, 2016.
302. Menon PR, Stapleton RD, McVeigh U, Rabinowitz T. Telemedicine as a tool to provide family conferences and palliative care consultations in critically ill patients at rural health care institutions: a pilot study. *Am J Hosp Palliat Care*. 2015;32(4):448-453.
303. Hennemann-Krause L, Lopes AJ, Araujo JA, Petersen EM, Nunes RA. The assessment of telemedicine to support outpatient palliative care in advanced cancer. *Palliat Support Care*. 2015;13(4):1025-1030.

304. Watanabe SM, Fairchild A, Pituskin E, Borgersen P, Hanson J, Fassbender K. Improving access to specialist multidisciplinary palliative care consultation for rural cancer patients by videoconferencing: report of a pilot project. *Support Care Cancer.* 2013;21(4):1201-1207.
305. Ostherr K, Killoran P, Shegog R, Bruera E. Death in the digital age: A systematic review of information and communication technologies in end-of-life care. *J Palliat Med.* 2016;19(4):408-420.
306. van Gurp J, van Selm M, Vissers K, van Leeuwen E, Hasselaar J. How outpatient palliative care teleconsultation facilitates empathic patient-professional relationships: a qualitative study. *PLoS One.* 2015;10(4):e0124387.
307. Sabesan S, Allen D, Caldwell P, et al. Practical aspects of telehealth: doctor-patient relationship and communication. *Intern Med J.* 2014;44(1):101-103.
308. Juckett G, Unger K. Appropriate use of medical interpreters. *Am Fam Physician.* 2014;90(7):476-480.
309. Silva MD, Genoff M, Zaballa A, et al. Interpreting at the end of life: A systematic review of the impact of interpreters on the delivery of palliative care services to cancer patients with limited english proficiency. *J Pain Symptom Manage.* 2016;51(3):569-580.
310. Lim FA, Bernstein I. Promoting awareness of LGBT issues in aging in a baccalaureate nursing program. *Nurs Educ Perspect.* 2012;33(3):170-175.
311. Candrian C, Lum H. Lesbian, gay, bisexual, and transgender communication. In: Wittenberg E, Ferrell BR, Goldsmith J, Smith T, Glajchen M, Handzo GF, eds. *Textbook of Palliative Care Communication.* New York, NY: Oxford University Press; 2015:229-237.
312. Bernat JL, Capron AM, Bleck TP, et al. The circulatory-respiratory determination of death in organ donation. *Crit Care Med.* 2010;38(3):963-970.
313. Prommer E. Organ donation and palliative care: can palliative care make a difference? *J Palliat Med.* 2014;17(3):368-371.
314. Robinson J, Thompson T. Transplantation and organ donation. In: Wittenberg E, Ferrell BR, Goldsmith J, Smith T, Glajchen M, Handzo GF, eds. *Textbook of Palliative Care Communication.* New York, NY: Oxford University Press; 2015:189-196.
315. Katzenbach JR, Smith DK. The discipline of teams. *Harv Bus Rev.* 1993;71(2):111-120.
316. Mount BM. Dealing with our losses. *J Clin Oncol.* 1986;4(7):1127-1134.
317. Cassell EJ. The nature of suffering and the goals of medicine. *N Engl J Med.* 1982;306(11):639-645.
318. Levy MH, Smith T, Alvarez-Perez A, et al. Palliative care, Version 1.2014. Featured updates to the NCCN Guidelines. *J Natl Compr Canc Netw.* 2014;12(10):1379-1388.
319. Health Care Financing Administration, US Department of Health and Human Services. Medicare program; hospice wage index. *Fed Regist.* 1997;62(153):42860-42883. 42 CFR §418. https://www.gpo.gov/fdsys/pkg/FR-1997-08-08/pdf/97-20775.pdf. Accessed May 1, 2017.
320. Cote T, Correoso-Thomas L, eds. *The Hospice Medical Director Manual.* 3rd ed. Chicago, IL: American Academy of Hospice and Palliative Medicine; 2016.
321. National Hospice Organization. *Standards of a Hospice Program of Care.* Arlington, VA: National Hospice Organization; 1993.
322. Thompson LL. *Making the Team: A Guide for Managers.* 2nd ed. Upper Saddle River, NJ: Pearson Prentice Hall; 2004.
323. Drinka TJK. Applying learning from self-directed work teams in business to curriculum development for interdisciplinary geriatric teams. *Educ Gerontol.* 1996;22(5):433-450.
324. Zeiss AM, Steffan AM. Interdisciplinary health care teams: the basic unit of geriatric care. In: Carstensen LL, Edelstein BA, Dornbrand L, eds. *The Practical Handbook of Clinical Gerontology.* Thousand Oaks, CA: Sage; 1996.

325. Lattanzi-Licht M. The hospice team: the wonder, worries, and work. *The Hospice Professional.* Arlington, VA: National Hospice Organization; 1996.
326. Drinka TJK. Interdisciplinary geriatric teams: approaches to conflict as indicators of potential to model teamwork. *Educ Gerontol.* 1994;20(1):87-103.
327. Julia MC, Thompson A. Essential elements of interprofessional teamwork. In: Casto RM, Julia MC, Ohio State University Commission on Interprofessional Education and Practice, eds. *Interprofessional Care and Collaborative Practice.* Belmont, CA: Wadsworth; 1994:43-57.
328. Larson CE, LaFasto FMJ. *Teamwork: What Must Go Right/What Can Go Wrong.* Newbury Park, CA: Sage; 1989.
329. Haugen DF, Friedemann N, Caraceni A. The interdisciplinary team. In: Hanks GWC, Cherny NI, Christakis NA, Fallon M, Kaasa S, Portenoy RK, eds. *Oxford Textbook of Palliative Medicine.* 4th ed. New York, NY: Oxford University Press; 2010:167-177.
330. Randall F, Downie RS. *Palliative Care Ethics: A Good Companion.* New York, NY: Oxford University Press; 1996.
331. West T. The interdisciplinary hospice team. Presented at: Seventh International Congress on Care of the Terminally Ill. 1990:Montreal.
332. Agar M, Luckett T. Outcome measures for palliative care research. *Curr Opin Support Palliat Care.* 2012;6(4):500-507.
333. Collins ES, Witt J, Bausewein C, Daveson BA, Higginson IJ, Murtagh FE. A systematic review of the use of the palliative care outcome scale and the support team assessment schedule in palliative care. *J Pain Symptom Manage.* 2015;50(6):842-853.e819.
334. Lowe JI, Herranen M. Interdisciplinary team. In: United States Health Resources Administration Division of Nursing, ed. *Hospice Education Program for Nurses.* Hyattsville, MD: US Department of Health and Human Services publication HRA 81-27; 1981:1047-1048.
335. Fan ET, Gruenfeld DH. When needs outweigh desires: the effects of resource interdependence and reward interdependence on group problem solving. *Basic Appl Soc Psychol.* 1998;20:45-56.
336. Jehn KA, Mannix EA. The dynamic nature of conflict: a longitudinal study of intragroup conflict and group performance. *Acad Manage J.* 2001;44(2):238-251.
337. Olivares Faundez V, Gil-Monte P, Miranda LM, Figueiredo-Ferraz H. Relationships between burnout and role ambiguity, role conflict, and employee absenteeism among health workers. *Terapia Psicologica.* 2014;32(2):111-120.
338. Johnson DW, Johnson FP. *Joining Together: Group Theory and Group Skills.* Upper Saddle River, NJ: Prentice Hall; 1975.
339. Lefton RE. The eight barriers to teamwork. *Personnel J.* 1988;67(1):18-21.
340. Forsyth D. *Group dynamics.* 2nd ed. Pacific Grove, CA: Brooks/Cole Publishing Company; 1990.
341. Gigone D, Hastie R. The common knowledge effect: information sharing and group judgment. *J Pers Soc Psychol.* 1993;65(5):959-974.
342. Gigone D, Hastie R. The impact of information on small group choice. *J Pers Soc Psychol.* 1993;72(1):132-140.
343. Mellor MJ, Hyer K, Howe JL. The geriatric interdisciplinary team approach: challenges and opportunities in educating trainees together from a variety of disciplines. *Educ Gerontol.* 2002;28(10):867-880.
344. O'Malley AS, Gourevitch R, Draper K, Bond A, Tirodkar MA. Overcoming challenges to teamwork in patient-centered medical homes: a qualitative study. *J Gen Intern Med.* 2015;30(2):183-192.
345. Mitchell R, Parker V, Giles M, Boyle B. The ABC of health care team dynamics: understanding complex affective, behavioral, and cognitive dynamics in interprofessional teams. *Health Care Manage Rev.* 2014;39(1):1-9.

346. Blackmore G, Persaud DD. Diagnosing and improving functioning in interdisciplinary health care teams. *Health Care Manag (Frederick)*. 2012;31(3):195-207.
347. Savel RH, Munro CL. Conflict management in the intensive care unit. *Am J Crit Care*. 2013;22(4):277-280.
348. Vorvick LJ, Avnon T, Emmett RS, Robins L. Improving teaching by teaching feedback. *Med Educ*. 2008;42(5):540-541.
349. Ende J. Feedback in clinical medical education. *JAMA*. 1983;250(6):777-781.
350. Stone D, Heen S. Thanks for the Feedback: The Science and Art of Receiving Feedback Well. New York, NY: Viking Penguin; 2014.
351. Thomas JD, Arnold RM. Giving feedback. *J Palliat Med*. 2011;14(2):233-239.
352. Kritek PA. Strategies for effective feedback. *Ann Am Thorac Soc*. 2015;12(4):557-560.
353. Sokol DK. Patients we don't like. *BMJ*. 2013;346:f3956.
354. Liaschenko J. Making a bridge: the moral work with patients we do not like. *J Palliat Care*. 1994;10(3):83-89.
355. Thurston A. A PIECE OF MY MIND. The unreasonable patient. *JAMA*. 2016;315(7):657-658.
356. Koh MY, Chong PH, Neo PS, et al. Burnout, psychological morbidity and use of coping mechanisms among palliative care practitioners: a multi-centre cross-sectional study. *Palliat Med*. 2015;29(7):633-642.
357. Slocum-Gori S, Hemsworth D, Chan WW, Carson A, Kazanjian A. Understanding compassion satisfaction, compassion fatigue and burnout: a survey of the hospice palliative care workforce. *Palliat Med*. 2013;27(2):172-178.
358. Jamieson L, Teasdale E, Richardson A, Ramirez A. The stress of professional caregivers. In: Hanks GWC, Cherny NI, Christakis NA, Fallon M, Kaasa S, Portenoy RK, eds. *Oxford Textbook of Palliative Medicine*. 4th ed. New York, NY: Oxford University Press; 2010:1445-1453.
359. White WL. Managing personal and organizational stress in the care of the dying. In: United States Health Resources Administration Division of Nursing, ed. *Hospice Education Program for Nurses*. Hyattsville, MD: US Department of Health and Human Services publication no. HRA 81-27; 1981.
360. Hudson FM. *The Adult Years: Mastering the Art of Self-Renewal*. San Francisco, CA: Jossey-Bass; 1991.
361. Makowski SK, Epstein RM. Turning toward dissonance: lessons from art, music, and literature. *J Pain Symptom Manage*. 2012;43(2):293-298.
362. Zambrano SC, Chur-Hansen A, Crawford GB. The experiences, coping mechanisms, and impact of death and dying on palliative medicine specialists. *Palliat Support Care*. 2014;12(4):309-316.
363. Hatem CJ. Renewal in the practice of medicine. *Patient Educ Couns*. 2006;62(3):299-301.
364. Frankl VE. Man's Search for Meaning: An Introduction to Logotherapy. 4th ed. Boston, MA: Beacon Press; 1992.
365. Chittenden EH, Ritchie CS. Work-life balancing: challenges and strategies. *J Palliat Med*. 2011;14(7):870-874.
366. Sanso N, Galiana L, Oliver A, Pascual A, Sinclair S, Benito E. Palliative care professionals' inner life: exploring the relationships among awareness, self-care, and compassion satisfaction and fatigue, burnout, and coping with death. *J Pain Symptom Manage*. 2015;50(2):200-207.
367. Beckman HB, Wendland M, Mooney C, et al. The impact of a program in mindful communication on primary care physicians. *Acad Med*. 2012;87(6):815-819.
368. Goodman MJ, Schorling JB. A mindfulness course decreases burnout and improves well-being among healthcare providers. *Int J Psychiatry Med*. 2012;43(2):119-128.
369. Mehta DH, Perez GK, Traeger L, et al. Building Resiliency in a Palliative Care Team: A Pilot Study. *J Pain Symptom Manage*. 2016;51(3):604-608.
370. Quill TE, Williamson PR. Healthy approaches to physician stress. *Arch Intern Med*. 1990;150(9):1857-1861.

371. Kearney MK, Weininger RB, Vachon ML, Harrison RL, Mount BM. Self-care of physicians caring for patients at the end of life: "being connected… a key to my survival". *JAMA.* 2009;301(11):1155-1164, E1151.
372. Estés CP. Women Who Run with the Wolves: Myths and Stories of the Wild Woman Archetype. New York, NY: Ballantine Books; 1992.
373. Nelson JE, Angus DC, Weissfeld LA, et al. End-of-life care for the critically ill: a national intensive care unit survey. *Crit Care Med.* 2006;34(10):2547-2553.
374. Rodriguez KL, Young AJ. Perspectives of elderly veterans regarding communication with medical providers about end-of-life care. *J Palliat Med.* 2005;8(3):534-544.
375. Rubenfeld GD, Curtis JR. End-of-life care in the intensive care unit: a research agenda. *Crit Care Med.* 2001;29(10):2001-2006.
376. Back AL, Arnold RM, Tulsky JA, Baile WF, Fryer-Edwards KA. Teaching communication skills to medical oncology fellows. *J Clin Oncol.* 2003;21(12):2433-2436.
377. Fallowfield L, Jenkins V, Farewell V, Saul J, Duffy A, Eves R. Efficacy of a cancer research UK communication skills training model for oncologists: a randomised controlled trial. *Lancet.* 2002;359(9307):650-656.
378. Yedidia MJ, Gillespie CC, Kachur E, et al. Effect of communications training on medical student performance. *JAMA.* 2003;290(9):1157-1165.
379. Bird J, Hall A, Maguire P, Heavy A. Workshops for consultants on the teaching of clinical communication skills. *Med Educ.* 1993;27(2):181-185.
380. Maguire P, Fairbairn S, Fletcher C. Consultation skills of young doctors: I-benefits of feedback training in interviewing as students persist. *Br Med J (Clin Res Ed).* 1986;292(6535):1573-1576.
381. Clay A, Ross E, Knudsen NW, Grochowski C. A breaking bad news exercise to assess student competence prior to graduation. *MedEdPORTAL Publications.* 2015:10015. https://www.mededportal.org/publication/10015. Accessed May 1, 2017.
382. Smyth P, Sim V. Objective structured clinical examination (OSCE) station on communicating poor prognosis to the family in a neurological acute care setting. *MedEdPORTAL Publications.* 2014;10:9700. https://www.mededportal.org/publication/9700. Accessed May 1, 2017.
383. Mintzer M, Chen A, Conway Cooper T, et al. Breaking bad news using role playing: a multimedia instructional activity for teaching medical trainees. *MedEdPORTAL Publications.* 2014;10:9798. https://www.mededportal.org/publication/9798. Accessed May 1, 2017.
384. Lichter I, Mooney J, Boyd M. Biography as therapy. *Palliat Med.* 1993;7(2):133-137.
385. Penderell A, Brazil K. The spirit of palliative practice: a qualitative inquiry into the spiritual journey of palliative care physicians. *Palliat Support Care.* 2010;8(4):415-420.

Index

AAHPM quality indicators, 5
abandonment
    fears of, 12, 30, 42
    palliative care issues, 83
    uncertainty about, 25t
access to care, communication barriers and, 16
accountability, IDTs, 104
acknowledgement of emotions, 38
advocacy, 82–83
affect, relationships and, 2
age, stress and, 119t
anger
    encounters with, 117
    fear and, 38
anxiety
    of hospice patients, 11
    lack of information and, 30–31
appetite, loss of, 75
Ask-Tell-Ask approach, 21, 24t, 40, 58
assumptions, listening barriers, 14–15
attention spans, listening and, 15
autocratic leaders, 104
autonomy
    enhanced, 72
    levels of, 54
    shared decision making and, 53
autopsies, 47

bad news. *see also* serious news
    communication of, 29–47
    death notifications, 46
    disclosure of, 11
    sharing, 6
bereavement, death notifications, 45–47
"best interest," description of, 72
body language, 37. *see also* nonverbal communication
body positioning, 19
burnout, 3, 117–118

care plans, 42
caregivers. *see also* families
    burnout, 117–118
    communication interventions and, 3
    patient denial and, 60–61
    of patients with dementia, 84–86
Center for Organ Recovery, 93–94
Centers for Medicare and Medicaid Services (CMS)
    on interdisciplinary teams, 97
    patient experience scores, 5
certainty, listening barriers, 14–15
chaplains, 12, 104
child life specialists, 87
children
    communication with, 87
    of dying parents, 87
clarification
    asking for, 106
    communication and, 23t
    giving feedback and, 115–116
    information sharing and, 21
clinicians. *see also* physician-patient interactions; physicians
    communication, 3–5
    fear of causing harm, 13
    physician fears, 13–14
    sense of personal achievement, 3
collaboration, decision making and, 53
colleagues
    communication with, 82–84
    giving feedback to, 115–116
    relationships with, 122t
College of American Pathologists, 47
communication, 1–7. *see also specific* issues
    barriers to, 9–18, 10t
    clinical situations, 31, 43
    clinician's, 3–5
    components of, 3
    effective, 1–3, 22t–23t
    general guidelines, 7t

communication *(continued)*
    ineffective, 4
    key tasks, 6
    lack of training, 14
    with loved ones, 65–79
    making contracts, 42
    nonverbal, 19–20
    patient-centered, 1–2
    problem-soving skills and, 106–107
    relationship-centered, 2
    of serious news, 29–47
    strategies, 19–27
    training, 3, 125–127, 125*t*, 126*t*
compassion, communication and, 6
confidentiality, rights to, 81–82
conflicts
    anticipation of, 75–76
    heated, 77
    interpersonal, 113*t*
    management of, 114–115
    mediating in, 75–76
    naming of, 112
    negotiation strategies, 76–77
    nontraditional families and, 90–93
    problem-based discussions, 105
    resolutions, 114–115
    role ambiguity and, 105–106
    types of, 105–106
    unresolved, 112*t*
confrontation, communication and, 23*t*
consultations, 82–84
consulting physicians, 85*t*–86*t*
contracts, making, 42
control, sense of, 42
coping
    with burnout, 117–118
    family fears, 12
    patient fears, 12
    prognostic awareness and, 62–64
    resources for, 120
    shared decision-making and, 6
    with stress, 117–125

costs
    interdisciplinary teams and, 97
    resource outcomes and, 3
counseling elements, 73–75
cultural factors
    access to care and, 16
    barriers to communication, 9–12, 10*t*
    communication and, 5
    communication of serious news and, 31
    information sharing, 11
    nonverbal communication and, 19
death
    child's understanding of, 87
    communication about, 32
    experience of, 11
    family responses to, 70–71
    patient fears of, 12
    physician's fear of, 13
death notifications, 45–47
decision makers
    anticipating conflicts, 75–76
    medical, 73
decision making
    clinical, 49–56
    clinical situations, 50–51, 55–56
    continuum of, 54*f*
    cultural barriers, 12
    facilitation of, 107
    family involvement in, 11
    interdisciplinary teams, 107–108
    lack of capacity for, 84–86
    methods of, 109*t*
    planning and, 42
    sample statements, 53*t*
    shared, 2–3, 49–56, 109
    team process for, 108*f*
    without patient participation, 71–73
deep breathing exercises, 120
dementia
    communication with caregivers, 84–86
    communication with patients, 84–86
    patient fears, 12

democratic leaders, 104
demography, access to care and, 16
denial, 60–62
depersonalization, 3
depression
    decision making and, 72
    group psychotherapy and, 12
    vocabulary of, 17
diagnoses, communication issues, 29
dignity, symptom control and, 12
dignity therapy, 21
disease severity, awareness and, 57–58
dying
    communication about, 32, 87–88
    experience of, 11
    patient fears of, 12
    patient support during, 87–88

eating, vocabulary of, 17
emergency departments (EDs), 82
emotional responses
    acknowledgement of, 38
    anticipation of, 13
    body language and, 37
    children of dying parents, 87
    cumulative grief and, 13
    death notifications to, 46
    expression of empathy and, 38–40
    information sharing and, 21
    intimacy patterns and, 71
    normalization of, 25t
    physician response to, 38
    physician's fear of eliciting, 13
    physician's fear of expressing, 13
    relationships and, 2
    REMAP processes, 52t
empathy
    communication and, 25
    communication of, 74t
    death notifications to, 46
    description of, 21
    displays of, 41t
    effective communication and, 3

empathy *(continued)*
    expressions of, 38–40
    physical contact and, 24
    REMAP processes, 52t
    SPIKES protocol, 33t
    visit length and, 24
end-of-life care
    anticipating conflicts, 75–76
    family conferences in, 65
    loss of appetite and, 75
    medical decision making and, 53
    patient interviews and, 6
    planning issues, 57–58
    quality indicators, 5
    religious and spiritual issues, 9, 11
enhanced autonomy, 72
environmental issues
    communication barriers, 16
    communication of bad news, 32
evaluation of others, 14
existential concerns, 12
eye contact, communication and, 19

facial expressions, communication and, 19
families. *see also* caregivers
    coalitions, 70
    communication interventions and, 3
    death notifications to, 45–47
    denial and, 61–62
    difficult encounters with, 117
    fears of, 12
    grieving process, 84
    inclusion of, 30f
    intimacy patterns, 71
    involvement in decision making, 11
    nontraditional, 90–93, 92t
    note taking by, 36
    pairs, 68
    palliative care providers and, 83
    patient denial and, 60–61
    of patients with dementia, 84–86
    problem-based discussions, 105
    response to death, 70–71

families *(continued)*
    response to terminal illnesses, 70–71
    roles in illness, 70
    rules in illness, 70–71
    sense of control by, 42
    subsystems, 68–70
    summarizing interviews, 42
    telecommunication with, 88
    therapeutic silences and, 41
    triangles, 68, 70
families of choice, 92t
family conferences, 65
    clinical situations, 65–66, 77–79
    communication techniques, 74t
    counseling techniques, 74t
    exploring faith in, 76t
    facilitation of, 71–73
    roadmaps for, 73–79
family goals, anticipating conflicts, 75–76
family interaction models
    closed, 68, 69t
    disengaged, 67–68
    enmeshed, 67–68
    open, 68, 69t
family life cycles, 67
family preferences, decision making, 49–51
family relationships, disintegration of, 71
family satisfaction, 4–5
family systems theory, 66–67
fears
    acknowledgement of, 74t
    anger and, 38
    clinical situation, 81–82
feedback, 115–116, 116t
feeding, vocabulary of, 17
feelings. *see also* emotional responses; grief; guilt feelings
    of guilt, 74t
    physician's, 40
    shared, 40
fidgeting, 20
filial responsibilities, 11
Final Gifts (Callanan and Kelley), 87–88

financial losses, 12
Frankl, Viktor, 119

gelotology, 26
goals
    identification of, 51
    reframing of, 51–53, 52
"good deaths," 5
grief
    acknowledgement of, 74t
    emotional distance and, 13
    patient decline and, 84
group psychotherapy, 12
guilt feelings
    acknowledgement of, 74t
    children of dying parents, 87
    support groups and, 84

harm, fear of causing, 13
healing, empathetic relationships and, 21
hearing losses, 15, 15t
Holyquest (Perrino), 26
home healthcare aides, 104
honest labeling, 23t
honesty
    death notifications to, 46
    ethics and, 62
hope
    maintenance of, 26
    patient's focus on, 42
    support for patients, 74
"hope and worry" skills, 62, 64t
hospice
    family grief and, 84
    interdisciplinary teams, 97
hospice and palliative medicine
    communication and, 5–7
    consulting physicians and, 85t–86t
    death notifications, 45–47
    information about, 16–17
    interdisciplinary team approach, 95–116
    team coordinators, 103
    team leaders, 103

Hospice and Palliative Nurses Association, 5
hospice patients, anxiety of, 11
Hudson, Frederic, 118
humor
    appropriate, 26–27
    emotional significance of, 26
    perspective and, 26
    spiritual significance of, 26
    as therapy, 27t

"I wish" statements, 39–40, 62, 64t
IDTs. *see* interdisciplinary teams (IDTs)
illnesses. *see also* terminal diagnoses
    labeling in, 29
    patient's cognitive perspective, 35t
    patient's emotional perspective, 35t
    patient's knowledge of, 34–35
    physician's fear of, 13
    uncertainty management in, 24–25
independence, decision making and, 53
information sharing
    ask-tell-ask approach, 21
    with children, 87
    clinical situations, 43–45
    communication barriers and, 16
    confidentiality and, 81–82
    cultural beliefs about, 11
    encouragement of, 21
    in hospice and palliative care settings, 6
    nondisclosure requests, 63t
    patient dignity and, 12
    patient satisfaction and, 5
    patient's desire for, 37
    patient's memory and, 38
    patient's perspective, 35–38
    pauses in, 37
    persons involved in, 32, 34
    prognostic awareness and, 57–58
    small steps, 36–37
    timing of, 37
    "warning shots," 36–37
informed refusals, 62
institutional factors, 31

institutional support, for IDTs, 100–101
intensive care units (ICUs)
    communication with, 82
    family conferences and, 65
    family satisfaction, 5
    lengths of stay, 3
interdisciplinary teams (IDTs)
    absenteeism, 113t
    advantages of, 98t
    approaches to care, 95–116
    barriers to effectiveness, 111t–112t
    brainstorming by, 107
    building of, 99–111
    camaraderie, 110–111
    characteristics of, 97–98, 101t
    clinical situations, 95–96, 107
    conflict management, 114–115
    confrontation phase, 100t
    death notifications to, 46
    description of, 98t
    developmental phases of, 98, 99t–100t
    disadvantages of, 98t
    dysfunctional, 112–114, 113t–114t
    effective leadership, 103–104
    empowerment, 110–111
    forming phase, 99t
    functions of, 96
    giving feedback, 115–116
    goals of, 101–102
    hospice requirements, 97
    institutional support for, 100–101
    interpersonal conflicts, 113t–114t
    isolation of, 113t
    moral distress among, 76
    norming phase, 99t
    norms of, 102–103
    openness to new ideas, 109–110
    problematic relationships between, 114t
    prognosis discussions and, 58–59
    role ambiguity, 105
    role conflicts, 105–106
    role overload, 106
    role recognition, 104–106

interdisciplinary teams (IDTs) *(continued)*
    scapegoating, 113t
    self-evaluation by, 110, 112t
    support by, 39–40
    synergy, 110–111
    threats to performance by, 111–116
    types of, 101–102
interest, communication of, 74t
interpreters, use of, 90, 91t
interviews
    communicating bad news, 32–34
    goal changes in, 6
    information sharing, 35–38
    summarizing in, 42
intimacy, relationships and, 118
intuition, humor and, 26
invitation, SPIKES protocol, 33t

judgement of others, 14
judgements, stress overload and, 117–118

knowledge
    fear of lacking, 14
    patient's, 34–35
    SPIKES protocol, 33t

laissez-faire leaders, 104
language barriers
    to effective communication, 10t
    information sharing and, 36
    limited English proficiency and, 17, 90
    medical language and, 16–17
    nonverbal cues and, 19
    use of interpreters, 90
    vocabulary, 17–18
laughter, benefits of, 26
leadership
    dysfunctional, 113t
    effective, 103–104
    promotional, 111t
    shared, 104
    skills, 103f
    styles of, 103–104

leads, communication and, 22t
lengths of stay, ICU, 3
LGBT patients, 90–93. *see also* non-heterosexual individuals
life events, stress and, 119t
listening
    barriers to, 10t, 14–15
    in family conferences, 74t
    to patients, 20–21
    patient's ability, 37
loneliness, patient's sense of, 30

malpractice litigation, 3
Managing Cancer and Living Meaningfully (CALM) protocol, 12
meaning, search for, 74t
"Measuring What Matters" tool, 5
medical language, 16–18
mindfulness techniques, 120
misconceptions, correction of, 38
mood, communication and, 3
motivation, stress and, 119t
multidisciplinary teams. *see* interdisciplinary teams (IDTs)

narrative medicine, 20–21
National Hospice and Palliative Care Organization, 97
negotiation strategies
    confidentiality and, 81–82
    conflict resolution, 76–77
New England Organ Bank, 93–94
non-heterosexual individuals, 92t, 93t. *see also* LGBT patients
nonabandonment, stress placed on, 42
nondisclosure requests, 63t
nonverbal communication, 19–20. *see also* body language
    death notifications to, 46
    emotional responses and, 37
    of pain, 86
    skills, 20t
NURSE mnemonic, 38, 39f, 43–45, 55–56
nurses, 32, 104
nutritional support, 75

oligarchic leaders, 104
organ donation, 93–94
organ procurement organizations (OPOs), 93–94
organizational barriers
    access to care, 16
    access to information, 16
    to effective communication, 10t
    environmental issues, 16
    lack of support, 16
    reimbursement issues, 16
    standards of performance and, 16
    stress and, 119t

pain
    alleviation of, 126
    emotional, 126
    nonverbal indicators of, 86
    patient's descriptions of, 14
    spiritual, 126
palliative care consultations, 82–83, 88
paraphrasing, communication and, 23t
paternalism, palliative, 54
patient-centered care, 1
patient-centered communications, 3t
patient expectations
    barriers to communication, 9
    information sharing and, 21
    listening and, 20–21
    wishes for knowledge, 35
patient goals, anticipating conflicts, 75–76
patient histories, review of, 96
patient perspectives
    eliciting, 35t
    identification of, 51
    information sharing, 35–38
patient preferences
    care as death approaches, 3
    communication of serious news, 30–31, 30t
    shared decision making, 49–51, 53–56
patient satisfaction, 4–5
patient-specific goals, 49–51

patients
    communication style of, 36
    in denial, 60–61
    difficult encounters with, 117
    fears of, 12
    goals of, 3
    knowledge assessment, 34–35
    narrative of, 20–21
    nonverbal communication by, 20
    note taking by, 36
    palliative care providers and, 83
    sense of control by, 42
    summarizing interviews, 42
    therapeutic silences and, 41
patronization, feelings and, 29
perception, SPIKES protocol, 33t
Perrino, Anthony, 26
personality, stress and, 119t
personhood, relationships and, 2
Pew-Fetzer Task Force on Advancing Psychosocial Health Education, 2
physical distance, 19
physician-patient interactions
    communication barriers, 13–15
    core function of communications, 4f
    counseling elements in, 73–75
    effective communication and, 16
    goals of, 1
    patient vulnerability and, 6
    satisfaction with, 117
    shared decision making and, 53
    sharing contact information, 42
    trust and, 11
    uncertainty management, 25
physicians
    burnout, 117–118
    communication tasks, 84–86
    distress of, 120
    needs of, 119–120
    psychological distress of, 120
    psychological issues for, 119–120

physicians *(continued)*
    role flexibility, 104
    signs of stress overload, 120t
    spiritual distress of, 120
    spiritual issues, 119–120
planning
    decision making and, 42
    prognostic awareness and, 57–58
pneumonia, in dementia, 84
posttraumatic stress disorder, 72
posture, 19
primary care physicians (PCPs), 32
problem-solving skills, IDTs, 106–107
process conflicts, 105
prognosis
    clinical situations, 43–45, 61
    communication of, 29, 57–64
    discussion of, 58–59
    information about, 38
    nondisclosure requests, 63t
    patient's desire for knowledge, 37
    patient's feelings about, 38
    troubleshooting, 62–64
prognostic awareness
    gauging, 57–58
    promotion of, 25
    troubleshooting, 62–64
psychological barriers
    to effective communication, 10t
    family fears, 12
    patient fears, 12
    physician fears, 13–14
purpose, support for patients, 74

quality of life
    communication issues and, 86
    effective communication and, 3
    group psychotherapy and, 12
questions
    keeping lists of, 42
    open-ended, 11–12, 22t, 54

reassurance, information sharing and, 21
referring providers, 82–84
reflection, communication and, 23t, 25
reimbursement issues, 16
relationship-centered care, 2, 21
relationships
    communication of serious news and, 31
    conflicts, 105
    intimacy and, 118
religion
    barriers to communication, 9, 11
    as source of conflicts, 76
REMAP processes, 52t
    clinical situation, 77–79
    family conferences and, 73
repetition strategies, 22t
resource allocations, 3
responsibilities, ODTs, 104
role ambiguity, 105
role difficulties, stress and, 119t

Saunders, Cicely, 120
SAVE mnemonic, 38, 39f
scapegoating, 70
self-awareness, 122t–124t
self-care, 122t–124t
self-disclosure, 40
sense of self, 95, 118
sensitivity, humor and, 26
serious news. *see also* bad news
    clinical situations, 43–45
    communication guidelines, 30–31
    communication of, 29–47
    communication protocol, 32–45
    note taking by stakeholders, 36
    "warning shots," 36
settings, SPIKES protocol, 33t
sexual orientations, 90–93, 92t
sexuality, communication about, 91–92
short message services (SMS), 88
side effects, patient fears, 12
silence, communication and, 20
social aspects of care, 5

social supports, stress and, 119t
social touch, 20
social workers
    clinical situation, 81–82
    hospice team, 87
    role flexibility, 104
societal values, 9
"some-other" technique, 62
SPIKES protocol, 32, 33t
    clinical situation, 77–79
    family conferences and, 73
spiritual issues, physician, 119–120
spiritual leaders, partnering with, 12
spirituality
    barriers to communication, 9, 11
    cultural issues, 12
    as source of conflicts, 76
stakeholders, SPIKES protocol, 33t
standards of performance, 16
stress
    coping with, 117–125
    lack of information and, 30–31
    management strategies, 118–125, 122t
    overload, 120t
    overload among physicians, 119t
substituted judgement, 72
suffering, sense of self and, 95
summarizing
    communication and, 23t, 25
    SPIKES protocol, 33t
support groups, 84
surrogates. *see also* caregivers
    communication interventions and, 3
    optimism bias, 58–59
    shared decision making, 50
survival, effective communication and, 3
sympathetic pain, 13
symptom control, patient dignity and, 12
systemic barriers
    access to care, 16
    access to information, 16
    to effective communication, 10t
    environmental issues, 16

systemic barriers (continued)
    lack of support, 16
    reimbursement issues, 16
    standards of performance and, 16
systemic factors, communication and, 31

task conflicts, 105
team paradox, 103
teamwork, effective, 100. *see also* interdisciplinary teams (IDTs)
telemedicine
    communication strategies, 88–89, 89t
    phone-based technology, 89t
    text-based technology, 89t
    video-based technology, 89t
tensing up, nonverbal communication by, 20
terminal diagnoses, 11. *see also* illnesses
terminal illnesses
    family responses to, 70–71
    hope maintained in, 26
    patient goals in, 87–88
therapeutic dialogue, 6
therapeutic humor, 27t
therapeutic regimens, adherence to, 3
therapeutic relationships, 13, 14
therapeutic silences, 41
touch, 19
    social, 20
training
    communication, 3
    communication skills, 125–127, 125t, 126t
    in communication skills, 14
treatment plans, 96
treatments, side effects, 12
troubleshooting prognosis, 62–64
trust, interactions and, 11

uncertainty
    labeling and, 29
    management of, 24–25, 25t
unreasonable behaviors, 60–61

vacations, need for, 118
validation
    of emotions, 38
    information sharing and, 21
values
    identification of, 51
    REMAP processes, 52t
    sense of self and, 118
    support for patients, 74
verbal following, communication and, 22t

vocabulary
    meanings and, 17–18
    problematic phrases, 17–18
    "warning shots," 36
voice, tone of, 19
vulnerability of patients, 6

"warning shots," 36, 46
"We" statements, 40